Carb Cycling Cookbook for Beginners

Revitalize Your Body & Mind. The Ultimate Carb-Cycling Blueprint for Weight Loss, Muscle Gain, and Peak Performance. Includes 45-Day Meal Plan

Mason T. Harlow

© Copyright 2024 by Mason T. Harlow All rights reserved.

The following book is provided below with the aim of delivering information that is as precise and dependable as possible. However, purchasing this book implies an acknowledgment that both the publisher and the author are not experts in the discussed topics, and any recommendations or suggestions contained herein are solely for entertainment purposes. It is advised that professionals be consulted as needed before acting on any endorsed actions.

This statement is considered fair and valid by both the American Bar Association and the Committee of Publishers Association, and it holds legal binding throughout the United States.

Moreover, any transmission, duplication, or reproduction of this work, including specific information, will be deemed an illegal act, regardless of whether it is done electronically or in print. This includes creating secondary or tertiary copies of the work or recorded copies, which are only allowed with the express written consent from the Publisher. All additional rights are reserved.

The information in the following pages is generally considered to be a truthful and accurate account of facts. As such, any negligence, use, or misuse of the information by the reader will result in actions falling solely under their responsibility. There are no scenarios in which the publisher or the original author can be held liable for any difficulties or damages that may occur after undertaking the information described herein.

Additionally, the information in the following pages is intended solely for informational purposes and should be considered as such. As fitting its nature, it is presented without assurance regarding its prolonged validity or interim quality. Mention of trademarks is done without written consent and should not be construed as an endorsement from the trademark holder.

TABLE OF CONTENTS

CHAPTER 1: INTRODUCTION TO CARB CYCLING 11
The Science Behind Carb Cycling 11
Benefits for Body and Mind 12
Debunking Common Myths 14

CHAPTER 2: SETTING UP FOR SUCCESS 17
Preparing Your Kitchen for Carb Cycling 17
Understanding Macronutrients 18

CHAPTER 3: HIGH-CARB DAY RECIPES 21
Breakfasts to Fuel Your Day 21
1. OATMEAL BANANA BERRY BAKE 21
2. SWEET POTATO AND BLACK BEAN BREAKFAST BURRITOS 21
3. MANGO CHIA PUDDING PARFAIT 22
4. PEANUT BUTTER AND JELLY OATMEAL 22
5. SPINACH AND FETA BREAKFAST QUICHE 23
6. BLUEBERRY ALMOND PANCAKES 24

Energizing Lunches 24
1. QUINOA POWER SALAD 24
2. SWEET POTATO LENTIL BOWL 25
3. CHICKPEA AVOCADO WRAP 26
4. TURKEY AND QUINOA STUFFED PEPPERS 26
5. ASIAN CHICKEN SALAD 27
6. MEDITERRANEAN LENTIL PASTA SALAD 27

Satisfying Dinners 28
1. ROASTED VEGETABLE AND FARRO BOWL 28
2. LEMON HERB CHICKEN PASTA 29
3. BALSAMIC GLAZED SALMON WITH QUINOA AND SPINACH 29
4. THAI PEANUT SWEET POTATO BUDDHA BOWL 30
5. MUSHROOM RISOTTO WITH PEAS 31
6. CREAMY COCONUT LENTIL CURRY 31

Snacks and Smoothies 32
1. TROPICAL GREEN SMOOTHIE 32
2. PEANUT BUTTER ENERGY BALLS 33
3. AVOCADO TOAST WITH TOMATO AND BASIL 33
4. CINNAMON APPLE CHIPS 34
5. BERRY BANANA SMOOTHIE BOWL 34
6. HUMMUS AND VEGGIE ROLL-UPS 34

CHAPTER 4: LOW-CARB DAY RECIPES 37

MORNING STARTERS 37
    1. SPINACH AND FETA OMELETTE 37
    2. ALMOND FLOUR PANCAKES 37
    3. AVOCADO AND EGG BREAKFAST BOWL 38
    4. COTTAGE CHEESE AND BERRY PARFAIT 38
    5. SMOKED SALMON AND CREAM CHEESE ROLL-UPS 39
    6. KETO AVOCADO CHOCOLATE SMOOTHIE 39

LIGHT AND FRESH LUNCHES 40
    1. GRILLED CHICKEN AND AVOCADO SALAD 40
    2. ZUCCHINI NOODLE CAPRESE 40
    3. CUCUMBER SHRIMP AVOCADO SALAD 41
    4. CAULIFLOWER RICE STIR-FRY WITH VEGETABLES 41
    5. GREEK CHICKEN SALAD 42
    6. BROCCOLI AND CHEESE STUFFED PEPPERS 42

HEARTY DINNERS 43
    1. HERB-CRUSTED SALMON WITH ASPARAGUS 43
    2. BEEF AND BROCCOLI STIR-FRY 44
    3. GRILLED PORK CHOPS WITH HERB BUTTER 44
    4. CAJUN SHRIMP AND AVOCADO SALAD 45
    5. TURKEY BACON WRAPPED ASPARAGUS 45
    6. SPICY KALE AND CHICKEN SOUP 46

LOW-CARB SNACKS AND TREATS 46
    1. CHEESY KALE CHIPS 46
    2. AVOCADO DEVILED EGGS 47
    3. CUCUMBER TUNA BOATS 47
    4. BAKED PEPPERONI CHIPS 48
    5. ALMOND BUTTER CELERY STICKS 48
    6. MINI BELL PEPPER NACHOS 49

CHAPTER 5: BALANCED MEALS FOR TRANSITION DAYS 51

NUTRIENT-RICH BREAKFASTS 51
    1. SUNRISE TURMERIC QUINOA BOWL 51
    2. GREEN GODDESS AVOCADO TOAST 51
    3. BERRY CHIA OVERNIGHT OATS 52
    4. SAVORY MUSHROOM AND SPINACH FRITTATA 52
    5. SMOKED SALMON BREAKFAST SALAD 53

BALANCED LUNCH OPTIONS 53
    1. ROASTED CHICKPEA AND QUINOA SALAD 53
    2. TURKEY AND AVOCADO WRAP 54
    3. SPINACH AND GOAT CHEESE STUFFED CHICKEN 54
    4. LEMON HERB TILAPIA OVER KALE AND QUINOA SALAD 55

WHOLESOME DINNERS 55

- 1. HERB-CRUSTED SALMON WITH LENTILS 55
- 2. STUFFED ACORN SQUASH 56
- 3. LEMON GARLIC SHRIMP WITH ZUCCHINI NOODLES 57
- 4. CREAMY MUSHROOM AND SPINACH RISOTTO 57

SNACKS FOR ENERGY BALANCE 58
- 1. CRUNCHY KALE CHIPS 58
- 2. ALMOND BUTTER ENERGY BITES 59
- 3. SPICY ROASTED CHICKPEAS 59
- 4. AVOCADO AND COTTAGE CHEESE STUFFED BELL PEPPERS 60
- 5. GREEK YOGURT AND BERRY PARFAIT 60
- 6. CUCUMBER HUMMUS BITES 60

CHAPTER 6: RECIPES FOR MUSCLE GAIN 63

PROTEIN-PACKED BREAKFASTS 63
- 1. SPINACH AND FETA PROTEIN MUFFINS 63
- 2. QUINOA AND EGG BREAKFAST BOWL 63
- 3. TURKEY SAUSAGE AND SWEET POTATO SKILLET 64
- 4. GREEK YOGURT OAT PANCAKES 64
- 5. CHICKEN AND EGG BREAKFAST BURRITO 65

POST-WORKOUT LUNCHES 65
- 1. GRILLED CHICKEN AND QUINOA SALAD 65
- 2. TUNA AND CHICKPEA PITA POCKETS 66
- 3. SWEET POTATO AND BLACK BEAN BURRITO BOWL 67
- 4. EGGS AND TURKEY BACON ON WHOLE GRAIN TOAST 67
- 5. PROTEIN-PACKED SMOOTHIE 68

MUSCLE-BUILDING DINNERS 68
- 1. BEEF AND BROCCOLI STIR-FRY 68
- 2. SALMON WITH QUINOA AND SPINACH SALAD 69
- 3. TURKEY MEATBALLS WITH SPAGHETTI SQUASH 69
- 4. GRILLED STEAK WITH SWEET POTATO FRIES 70

RECOVERY SNACKS 71
- 1. COTTAGE CHEESE AND PEAR PARFAIT 71
- 2. AVOCADO CHOCOLATE MOUSSE 71
- 3. GREEK YOGURT WITH HOMEMADE GRANOLA 71
- 4. PROTEIN PEANUT BUTTER BANANA SMOOTHIE 72
- 5. SWEET POTATO PROTEIN BROWNIES 72
- 6. ALMOND JOY PROTEIN BALLS 73

CHAPTER 7: FAT LOSS-FOCUSED RECIPES 75

METABOLISM-BOOSTING BREAKFASTS 75
- 1. SPICY AVOCADO TOAST WITH EGG 75
- 2. GREEN TEA SMOOTHIE BOWL 75

- 3. CINNAMON AND OATMEAL PROTEIN PANCAKES 76
- 4. TURMERIC SCRAMBLED EGGS 76
- 5. GRAPEFRUIT AND AVOCADO SALAD 77

Fat-Burning Lunches 77
- 1. SPINACH AND CHICKEN SALAD WITH AVOCADO DRESSING 77
- 2. TURMERIC LENTIL SOUP 78
- 3. GRILLED SALMON WITH MANGO SALSA 78
- 4. SPICY CHICKPEA AND QUINOA BOWL 79
- 5. ZUCCHINI NOODLES WITH PESTO AND CHERRY TOMATOES 79

Light and Lean Dinners 80
- 1. GRILLED TILAPIA WITH LEMON HERB QUINOA 80
- 2. VEGGIE STUFFED BELL PEPPERS 80
- 3. BAKED COD WITH SPINACH AND TOMATOES 81
- 4. SPICY SHRIMP AND ZUCCHINI NOODLES 82

Low-Calorie Snacks 82
- 1. CUCUMBER ROLL-UPS WITH HUMMUS 82
- 2. GREEK YOGURT AND BERRY CUPS 83
- 3. CHILLED AVOCADO SOUP SHOTS 83
- 4. CARROT AND ZUCCHINI MINI MUFFINS 84
- 5. SPICY ROASTED CHICKPEAS 84
- 6. WATERMELON CUCUMBER BITES 85

CHAPTER 8: VEGETARIAN AND VEGAN OPTIONS 87

Plant-Based High-Carb Meals 87
- 1. QUINOA AND BLACK BEAN BURRITO BOWL 87
- 2. VEGAN LENTIL BOLOGNESE 87
- 3. SWEET POTATO AND CHICKPEA CURRY 88
- 4. HIGH-CARB VEGAN PIZZA 88

Low-Carb Vegetarian Delights 89
- 1. ZUCCHINI NOODLES WITH AVOCADO PESTO 89
- 2. CAULIFLOWER RICE STIR-FRY 90
- 3. MUSHROOM AND SPINACH OMELETTE 90

Vegan Snacks and Desserts 91
- 1. VEGAN CHOCOLATE AVOCADO TRUFFLES 91
- 2. VEGAN BANANA NUT MUFFINS 91
- 3. CRISPY KALE CHIPS 92

CHAPTER 9: QUICK AND EASY RECIPES 93

15-Minute Breakfasts 93
- 1. AVOCADO TOAST WITH POACHED EGG 93
- 2. BERRY AND YOGURT SMOOTHIE 93
- 3. SPINACH AND FETA MICROWAVE MUG OMELETTE 94

QUICK LUNCHES FOR BUSY DAYS 94
    1. CHICKPEA SALAD SANDWICH 94
    2. AVOCADO & QUINOA SALAD 95
    3. TURKEY & SPINACH WRAP 95
SPEEDY DINNERS 96
    1. PAN-SEARED SALMON WITH AVOCADO SALSA 96
    2. CHICKPEA AND SPINACH STIR-FRY 96
    3. QUICK VEGGIE PASTA 97
SIMPLE SNACKS 97
    1. APPLE SLICES WITH PEANUT BUTTER 97
    2. GREEK YOGURT AND HONEY PARFAIT 98
    3. HUMMUS AND VEGGIE STICKS 98

CHAPTER 10: THE 45-DAY CARB CYCLING MEAL PLAN **99**

WEEK 1-6: DAILY MEAL PLANS 99
ADJUSTING THE PLAN TO YOUR NEEDS 100
TRACKING YOUR PROGRESS 102
MEASUREMENT CONVERSION TABLE 104

CHAPTER 11: BEYOND THE PLATE **105**

COMPLEMENTING CARB CYCLING WITH EXERCISE 105
MINDFULNESS AND MENTAL HEALTH..106
BUILDING A SUPPORTIVE COMMUNITY 107

CHAPTER 1: INTRODUCTION TO CARB CYCLING
THE SCIENCE BEHIND CARB CYCLING

In the heart of every fitness enthusiast's journey lies the quest for the optimal diet—one that not only promises weight loss and muscle gain but also aligns with the hustle and bustle of daily life. Amidst the sea of dietary advice, carb cycling emerges as a beacon, guiding us through the fog with its flexible approach to eating. But what is the science behind carb cycling, and how can it catalyze our journey towards achieving peak physical and mental wellness? Let's dive deep into the realms of biology and nutrition to uncover the foundation upon which carb cycling stands. Carb cycling is a dietary strategy that alternates between high-carb days and low-carb days. This approach is not merely a random oscillation between carb consumption but a thoughtful method grounded in our body's metabolic processes. To understand its efficacy, we need to explore how our bodies process carbohydrates and the hormonal symphony that orchestrates our metabolism. Carbohydrates, our body's preferred source of energy, are broken down into glucose during digestion. Glucose, in turn, fuels our daily activities and supports our brain function. The pancreas plays a pivotal role in managing our blood glucose levels through the secretion of two critical hormones: insulin and glucagon. On high-carb days, the increased intake of carbohydrates leads to a rise in blood glucose levels, prompting the pancreas to release insulin. Insulin facilitates the uptake of glucose by our muscles and liver, storing it as glycogen for future energy needs. This process is not just about fuel storage; it's about optimizing our body's ability to perform and recover, particularly after rigorous exercise. Conversely, low-carb days trigger a different metabolic pathway. With reduced carbohydrate intake, our body turns to stored fat for energy, a process known as ketosis. During this phase, the pancreas secretes glucagon, which signals the liver to convert stored glycogen and fat into glucose. This shift not only aids in fat loss but also teaches our body to become more efficient in fuel selection, enhancing our metabolic flexibility. But carb cycling's benefits extend beyond the physiological. This dietary approach harmonizes with our body's natural rhythms and lifestyle demands. Consider high-carb days as the tide that floods our muscles with energy, perfectly timed with our most strenuous workouts. These are the days when we harness the power of carbohydrates to fuel our performance and recovery. Low-carb days, on the other hand, are the ebb, a period of metabolic recalibration where our body turns to fat as its primary energy source, promoting weight loss and improving insulin sensitivity. This strategic alternation between fuel sources does more than just enhance our physical capabilities; it fosters a deeper connection with our body's signals. Carb cycling encourages us to attune to our hunger cues, energy levels, and performance fluctuations, transforming the way we approach eating from a rigid regimen to a dynamic dialogue with our body.

Moreover, carb cycling stands as a testament to the principle of balance. It acknowledges that no single diet fits all and that our nutritional needs fluctuate with our daily activities, stress levels, and fitness goals. This flexibility is particularly empowering for those who have felt constrained by the strictures of traditional diets. Carb cycling offers a path that accommodates social dinners, celebratory treats, and the occasional indulgence, reinforcing the idea that a healthy diet is not about deprivation but about sustainable choices that support our lifestyle. Critics of carb cycling argue that its effectiveness is merely anecdotal, lacking the robust evidence base that underpins other dietary approaches. While it's true that the realm of nutrition science is ever-evolving, with new studies continually shedding light on the intricacies of our metabolism, the anecdotal successes of carb cycling cannot be dismissed. These stories speak to the adaptability and resilience of our bodies, and to the power of a diet that respects our biological uniqueness. Carb cycling also opens the door to a more nuanced understanding of carbohydrates. Not all carbs are created equal, and this dietary approach encourages us to choose nutrient-dense sources—whole grains, fruits, and vegetables—that offer vitamins, minerals, and fiber. This shift in perspective is crucial, moving us away from the vilification of carbohydrates to a more holistic view of nutrition where quality and timing are key. As we embark on the carb cycling journey, it's essential to approach it with curiosity and patience. Our bodies are complex systems, and finding the right balance takes time and experimentation. It's about listening to our body's responses, adjusting our carb intake to align with our energy needs and fitness goals, and most importantly, embracing the process with kindness and flexibility. In essence, the science behind carb cycling is a dance between biology and lifestyle, a marriage of metabolic pathways and personal preferences. It offers a way to navigate the complexities of nutrition with grace, empowering us to make choices that fuel our bodies and enrich our lives. As we peel back the layers of scientific jargon, what emerges is a simple, yet profound truth: that in the rhythm of high and low, there's a harmony that resonates with the very essence of well-being.

BENEFITS FOR BODY AND MIND

The benefits of carb cycling extend far beyond the scales and gym performance; they touch upon every facet of our being, fostering a holistic sense of health that is both empowering and enlightening. At its core, carb cycling aligns with our body's innate rhythms, optimizing energy use and enhancing our physical health in a myriad of ways. This dance between high-carb and low-carb days not only fuels our workouts but also ignites our body's metabolic flexibility. By alternating our carbohydrate intake, we teach our bodies to efficiently switch between burning carbs and fats for fuel, a skill that can significantly improve our metabolic health. For those of us aiming to sculpt our physique, carb cycling proves to be a powerful ally. High-carb days support muscle growth by replenishing glycogen stores, a critical energy reserve for intense workouts, and aiding in recovery. On the flip side, low-carb days help in fat loss by encouraging the body to tap into fat stores for energy, leading to a leaner composition without sacrificing muscle mass. But the benefits are not confined to aesthetics or performance alone. Carb cycling has a profound impact on insulin sensitivity, a key marker of metabolic health. By moderating our carb intake, we can prevent the insulin spikes associated with constant high-carb diets, reducing the risk of developing insulin resistance—a precursor to diabetes and other metabolic disorders. The impact of carb cycling on mental wellness is equally remarkable. The brain, a voracious consumer of glucose, responds positively to the ebb and flow of carbohydrate availability. High-carb days can enhance mood and cognitive function by ensuring an ample supply of glucose, while low-carb days, by promoting ketosis, can lead to increased levels of beta-hydroxybutyrate, a ketone body known for its neuroprotective effects. This rhythmic dietary approach also teaches us to listen to our bodies, fostering a mindfulness that extends beyond mealtime. By paying attention to how our bodies respond to different macronutrient ratios, we cultivate a deeper connection with our physical and mental states, leading to more informed and intuitive eating practices. This mindfulness, a byproduct of the carb cycling journey, can enhance our overall sense of well-being, reducing stress and anxiety associated with food choices and dieting. Carb cycling's flexible nature also means it can be seamlessly woven into the social fabric of our lives. Unlike more restrictive diets, carb cycling accommodates the ebb and flow of social engagements and celebrations. This adaptability not only makes it a sustainable approach to nutrition but also ensures that our diet enriches rather than detracts from our social well-being. By eliminating the stress and guilt often associated with navigating diet restrictions in social settings, carb cycling allows us to enjoy life's pleasures while staying aligned with our health goals. Embarking on a carb cycling plan is an act of empowerment. It requires us to take charge of our diet, to make conscious decisions about our food intake based on our body's needs and our personal goals. This sense of autonomy is liberating, providing us with the tools to craft a diet that's uniquely tailored to our lifestyle. In doing so, we move away from the one-size-fits-all diets that dominate the nutritional landscape, embracing a more personalized approach to health and wellness. In the grand scheme of things, carb cycling is more than just a dietary strategy; it's a blueprint for a balanced life. It acknowledges the complex interplay between our physical and mental health, recognizing that true wellness is achieved not by extreme measures but through balance and flexibility. This harmony between body and mind is the cornerstone of a sustainable health journey, one that allows us to thrive not just in the present but for years to come. In a world where dietary advice is often contradictory and confusing, carb cycling stands out for its simplicity and effectiveness. It doesn't promise a quick fix but offers a sustainable path to health that respects our body's natural processes and our need for a diet that fits our unique lives.

DEBUNKING COMMON MYTHS

In the realm of nutrition, myths and misconceptions abound, clouding our understanding and often leading us astray. Carb cycling, despite its many benefits, has not been immune to this phenomenon. It's time to clear the air, to shine a light on the facts, and to debunk some of the most common myths surrounding this dietary strategy. By doing so, we empower ourselves with knowledge, stepping into a more informed relationship with our bodies and our plates.

Myth 1: Carb Cycling Is Overly Complex and Only Suitable for Athletes

One of the most pervasive myths about carb cycling is that it's an intricate science, tailor-made for the elite athlete. This couldn't be further from the truth. Yes, carb cycling does involve varying your carbohydrate intake across different days, but this practice is grounded in the natural rhythms of our bodies. It's a flexible approach that can be adapted to fit the lifestyle and goals of anyone looking to improve their health, whether you're a busy parent, a professional juggling deadlines, or someone taking their first steps into a more active life. Carb cycling is about listening to your body and responding to its needs—a practice that's as simple as it is profound.

Myth 2: Carb Cycling Will Leave You Feeling Depleted on Low-Carb Days

Another common concern is the fear of energy depletion on low-carb days. It's a valid concern, given that carbohydrates are our body's primary energy source. However, this fear overlooks the body's remarkable adaptability. On low-carb days, our bodies tap into alternative energy sources, such as fat stores, providing us with a sustained energy release. Many find that after an initial adjustment period, they experience more stable energy levels and even improved mental clarity on low-carb days, debunking the myth that these days are synonymous with fatigue.

Myth 3: Carb Cycling Is Just Another Fad Diet

In a world where new diets emerge and fade with the seasons, it's easy to lump carb cycling in with the latest nutritional fads. However, carb cycling is not a trend but a strategic approach to eating that aligns with our metabolic processes. It's based on the understanding that our bodies respond differently to nutrients at different times, influenced by our activity levels, hormonal changes, and overall health. By leveraging this knowledge, carb cycling offers a sustainable approach to nutrition that can be tailored to support long-term health goals, distinguishing it from the quick fixes and miracle diets that populate our social feeds.

Myth 4: Carb Cycling Means Saying Goodbye to Your Favorite Foods

One of the most discouraging myths is the belief that carb cycling requires giving up the foods you love. On the contrary, carb cycling is about balance and timing. It encourages a healthy relationship with food, where carbohydrates are not demonized but strategically enjoyed. High-carb days allow for the inclusion of whole grains, fruits, and even the occasional treat, ensuring that your diet remains varied and satisfying. Rather than imposing strict prohibitions, carb cycling promotes mindful eating, making room for your favorite foods within a structured, health-focused framework.

Myth 5: Carb Cycling Doesn't Support Long-Term Weight Management

Critics often claim that carb cycling is ineffective for long-term weight management, suggesting it offers only temporary results. This myth fails to consider the holistic benefits of carb cycling, which extends beyond simple weight loss. By improving metabolic flexibility, enhancing insulin sensitivity, and fostering a mindful approach to eating, carb cycling lays the groundwork for sustainable health improvements. It's not just about shedding pounds; it's about building a lifestyle that supports your body's needs, paving the way for lasting change.

Myth 6: Carb Cycling Is Incompatible With a Social Life

Lastly, there's the myth that carb cycling is too rigid to accommodate social events and dining out. This couldn't be further from the truth. The flexibility at the heart of carb cycling means it can be easily adjusted to fit social occasions. Planning high-carb days around events or choosing lower-carb options when dining out are simple strategies that ensure your social life and dietary goals can coexist harmoniously. Rather than isolating you, carb cycling can enhance your social experiences, providing a framework that supports enjoyment and health in equal measure. In debunking these myths, we open the door to a more nuanced understanding of carb cycling. It's a testament to the power of informed choice and the importance of questioning the myths that cloud our path to wellness. Armed with knowledge, we can navigate the nutritional landscape with confidence, embracing carb cycling not as a restrictive diet but as a flexible, empowering approach to eating that supports our body, mind, and spirit.

CHAPTER 2: SETTING UP FOR SUCCESS
PREPARING YOUR KITCHEN FOR CARB CYCLING

The essence of preparing your kitchen for carb cycling lies in adopting a philosophy of balance, variety, and readiness. It's about ensuring that you have the right ingredients and tools at hand to effortlessly switch between high-carb and low-carb days without falling into monotony or frustration. This preparation is not just physical but also mental, as it requires you to view your kitchen as a partner in your health journey—a space that is flexible, supportive, and inspiring. Imagine your kitchen as a stage set for two acts: the high-carb days that energize and replenish, and the low-carb days that focus on fat burning and mindfulness. To play these roles to perfection, your pantry needs to be versatile. For the high-carb days, stock up on whole grains like quinoa, brown rice, and oats. These are not just sources of carbohydrates but also rich in fiber, which aids digestion and keeps you feeling full. Sweet potatoes, legumes, and fresh fruits are other staples that provide energy and a burst of nutrients. Conversely, for your low-carb days, focus on high-quality proteins and fats. Eggs, chicken, fish, and lean cuts of beef become your main actors, supported by a cast of healthy fats like avocados, nuts, seeds, and olive oil. Leafy greens and low-carb vegetables such as broccoli, cauliflower, and zucchini should fill your fridge, ready to add volume and nutrients to your meals without the carb load. Meal prepping is your script for success in carb cycling. It's the practice that ensures you stay on track, regardless of the day's macro requirements. Begin by planning your meals for the week, considering the balance between high-carb and low-carb days. Cooking in bulk and storing meals in portion-controlled containers can save you time and decision fatigue during the week. Investing in a set of reliable kitchen scales and measuring cups can make meal prep more efficient and accurate, helping you keep track of your macronutrient intake. Remember, carb cycling is as much about the quantity of carbs as it is about their quality. A carb-cycling kitchen thrives on flexibility. This means having a variety of spices, herbs, and condiments at your disposal to keep meals interesting and flavorful. Experimenting with different cuisines can bring diversity to your diet, making each meal an opportunity to explore new tastes and textures. This culinary curiosity not only enhances the pleasure of eating but also ensures that your diet remains rich in a variety of nutrients. Just as a craftsman is only as good as his tools, your success in carb cycling can be enhanced by the quality of your kitchen equipment. A high-powered blender is indispensable for smoothies and soups, while a good set of knives makes meal prep a breeze. Slow cookers and pressure cookers are valuable allies, capable of producing flavorful, nutrient-dense meals with minimal effort. Beyond the physical preparation, setting up your kitchen for carb cycling involves a mental shift. It's about viewing your kitchen as a space of possibility, where creativity and health go hand in hand. This mindset shift is crucial for making carb cycling a sustainable part of your life, not just a temporary diet. Lastly, consider how your kitchen environment affects your eating habits. Is it inviting and organized, or cluttered and chaotic? A kitchen that's set up for success is one that encourages healthy eating through organization and accessibility. This might mean having fruits and vegetables visible and within easy reach, or setting up a dedicated space for meal prepping. Preparing your kitchen for carb cycling is not a one-time task but an ongoing process of adaptation and discovery. As you become more attuned to your body's needs and preferences, your kitchen setup will evolve. This adaptability is not just a response to practical needs but a reflection of the transformative journey that carb cycling represents.

UNDERSTANDING MACRONUTRIENTS

Macronutrients are the cornerstone of any diet, but in the world of carb cycling, they hold the key to unlocking your body's fullest potential. By demystifying these essential nutrients—carbohydrates, proteins, and fats—we can tailor our intake to harmonize with our body's rhythms and health goals, setting the stage for a transformative journey. Carbohydrates are often viewed through a simplistic lens—either vilified as the cause of weight gain or celebrated as the body's main energy source. The truth, however, lies in their complexity. Carbohydrates serve as the primary fuel for our brains and muscles, playing a crucial role in our overall energy levels and performance. They are stored in the muscles and liver as glycogen, ready to be mobilized during physical activity. Yet, not all carbs are created equal. There's a vast difference between the quick-release energy found in processed sugars and the slow, sustaining power of complex carbohydrates found in whole grains, fruits, and vegetables. Understanding this distinction is crucial in carb cycling, as it allows us to select carbs that support our energy needs on high-carb days and manage our intake on low-carb days, ensuring a balance that supports our body's metabolic health. Proteins, made up of amino acids, are the building blocks of our muscles, skin, enzymes, and hormones. They play a pivotal role in muscle repair and growth, making them a critical component of any diet, especially for those engaged in regular physical activity. In the context of carb cycling, protein intake remains relatively consistent, providing the body with the necessary nutrients to repair and build muscle tissue, irrespective of the day's carb intake. Incorporating a variety of protein sources, from lean meats and fish to legumes and dairy, ensures a comprehensive profile of essential amino acids. This diversity not only supports physical health but also adds a rich tapestry of flavors and textures to our meals, making the carb cycling experience both nutritious and enjoyable. Fats have long been misunderstood, often labeled as the dietary villain. Yet, they are essential to our health, involved in hormone production, nutrient absorption, and providing a concentrated source of energy. Fats also play a critical role in satiety, helping us feel full and satisfied after meals. In the world of carb cycling, fats become particularly important on low-carb days, providing the body with an alternative energy source when carbohydrates are limited. Emphasizing healthy fats from sources like avocados, nuts, seeds, and olive oil can enhance our overall health, contributing to cardiovascular health and reducing inflammation. Understanding macronutrients allows us to see the bigger picture—how they interact and complement each other within the framework of carb cycling. It's not just about adjusting carb intake but about finding the optimal balance of all three macronutrients to support our energy needs, workout performance, and recovery processes. This balance is dynamic, changing with our daily activities, energy expenditure, and personal health goals.

Practical Tips for Navigating Macronutrients

1. **Educate Yourself on Food Sources**: Learn which foods are high in carbohydrates, proteins, and fats. Understanding this will help you make informed decisions about your meals, ensuring a balanced intake of all three macronutrients.
2. **Listen to Your Body**: Pay attention to how your body responds to different macronutrient ratios. Some may thrive on higher carb days, while others might feel better with a higher proportion of fats and proteins. This process is personal and requires patience and attention.
3. **Keep a Food Diary**: Initially, tracking your intake of carbs, proteins, and fats can provide valuable insights into your eating habits and help you adjust your diet to better meet your carb cycling goals.
4. **Plan Your Meals**: Planning is crucial in carb cycling. Align your carb intake with your activity levels, planning higher carb meals on workout days and focusing on proteins and fats during rest or low-intensity days.
5. **Embrace Variety**: Incorporate a wide range of foods from all macronutrient groups to ensure you're getting a broad spectrum of nutrients. This not only supports your physical health but also keeps your meals exciting and flavorful. Understanding macronutrients is like acquiring the keys to a treasure chest of health and performance. It empowers us to navigate the carb cycling journey with confidence, making informed choices that align with our body's needs and our personal goals. This knowledge transforms our diet from a rigid plan to a dynamic, responsive dialogue with our body, enabling us to achieve balance, wellness, and vitality.

CHAPTER 3: HIGH-CARB DAY RECIPES

BREAKFASTS TO FUEL YOUR DAY

1. OATMEAL BANANA BERRY BAKE

P.T.: 10 min
C.T.: 30 min
M.C.: Baking
SERVINGS: 6
INGR.:
2 cups rolled oats
1 tsp baking powder
1/2 tsp salt
1 tsp cinnamon
1/4 cup maple syrup
2 cups almond milk
1 tsp vanilla extract
1 large ripe banana, sliced
1 cup mixed berries (blueberries, raspberries, strawberries)
1/2 cup chopped walnuts
DIRECTIONS:
Preheat oven to 375°F (190°C).
In a large bowl, mix oats, baking powder, salt, and cinnamon.
Stir in maple syrup, almond milk, and vanilla extract until well combined.
Fold in banana slices and half of the berries.
Pour mixture into a greased baking dish. Top with remaining berries and chopped walnuts.
Bake for 30 minutes, or until the top is golden and the oats are set.
TIPS:
Serve warm with a dollop of Greek yogurt for extra protein.
Leftovers can be stored in the refrigerator and reheated for a quick breakfast.
N.V.: Calories: 270, Fat: 8g, Carbs: 44g, Protein: 6g, Sugar: 15g

2. SWEET POTATO AND BLACK BEAN BREAKFAST BURRITOS

P.T.: 20 min
C.T.: 25 min
M.C.: Sautéing & Wrapping
SERVINGS: 4
INGR.:
2 medium sweet potatoes, peeled and diced
1 Tbsp olive oil
1 tsp cumin
1/2 tsp smoked paprika
Salt and pepper to taste
1 can black beans, drained and rinsed
4 large whole wheat tortillas
1 avocado, sliced
1/4 cup fresh cilantro, chopped
1/2 cup shredded cheddar cheese
4 Tbsp salsa
DIRECTIONS:
Preheat a skillet over medium heat and add olive oil and sweet potatoes.
Season with cumin, smoked paprika, salt, and pepper. Cook until tender, about 15 minutes.
Add black beans to the skillet and cook until

heated through.

Warm tortillas according to package instructions.

Assemble the burritos by dividing the sweet potato and bean mixture, avocado slices, cilantro, cheese, and salsa among the tortillas. Fold in the sides and roll up tightly.

TIPS:

For a crispy finish, place the rolled burritos in a skillet and cook until golden on each side.

Customize with your favorite toppings like sour cream, hot sauce, or scrambled eggs.

N.V.: Calories: 450, Fat: 15g, Carbs: 67g, Protein: 14g, Sugar: 8g

3. MANGO CHIA PUDDING PARFAIT

P.T.: 15 min (plus overnight soaking)
C.T.: 0 min
M.C.: Refrigeration
SERVINGS: 4
INGR.:

1/4 cup chia seeds

1 cup coconut milk

2 Tbsp honey

1 tsp vanilla extract

1 mango, diced

1/2 cup granola

DIRECTIONS:

In a bowl, mix chia seeds, coconut milk, honey, and vanilla extract. Stir well until combined.

Cover and refrigerate overnight, or until the chia seeds have absorbed the liquid and the mixture has thickened.

Layer the chia pudding with diced mango and granola in glasses to serve as parfaits.

TIPS:

Top with additional fruits like kiwi or pineapple for extra flavor and color.

For a crunchier texture, add more granola on top before serving.

N.V.: Calories: 290, Fat: 14g, Carbs: 38g, Protein: 5g, Sugar: 22g

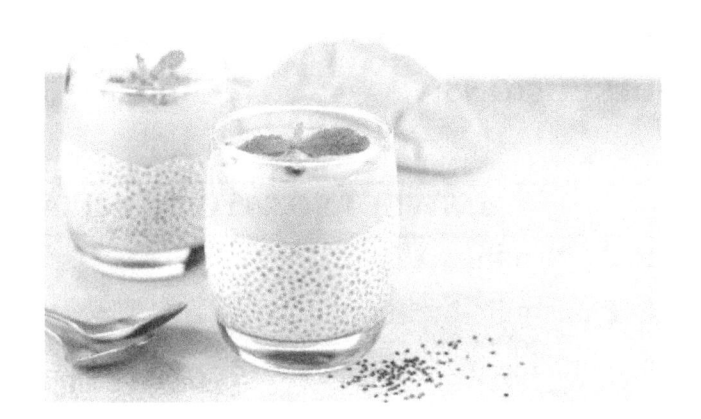

4. PEANUT BUTTER AND JELLY OATMEAL

P.T.: 5 min
C.T.: 10 min
M.C.: Boiling
SERVINGS: 2
INGR.:

1 cup rolled oats

2 cups water or milk

1 pinch salt

2 Tbsp natural peanut butter

2 Tbsp jelly or jam of choice

1 banana, sliced

1 Tbsp chia seeds

DIRECTIONS:

In a medium saucepan, bring water or milk to a boil. Add oats and salt, stirring occasionally, and cook until the oats are soft and have absorbed most of the liquid, about 5-7 minutes.

Remove from heat and stir in peanut butter and jelly until evenly mixed.

Serve hot, topped with banana slices and a sprinkle of chia seeds.

TIPS:

For added sweetness, drizzle with honey or maple syrup.

Use almond butter or cashew butter as a tasty alternative to peanut butter.

N.V.: Calories: 380, Fat: 14g, Carbs: 56g, Protein: 12g, Sugar: 20g

5. SPINACH AND FETA BREAKFAST QUICHE

P.T.: 15 min
C.T.: 35 min
M.C.: Baking
SERVINGS: 6
INGR.:

1 pre-made pie crust

5 eggs

1/2 cup milk

1 cup fresh spinach, chopped

1/2 cup feta cheese, crumbled

1/4 cup red onion, finely chopped

Salt and pepper to taste

1 tomato, sliced for topping

DIRECTIONS:

Preheat oven to 375°F (190°C).

Place the pie crust in a pie dish. Prick the bottom with a fork to prevent bubbling.

In a mixing bowl, whisk together eggs, milk, salt, and pepper.

Stir in spinach, feta cheese, and red onion.

Pour the mixture into the pie crust.

Arrange tomato slices on top.

Bake in the preheated oven for 35 minutes, or until the quiche is set and the crust is golden brown.

TIPS:

Let the quiche cool for a few minutes before slicing for cleaner cuts.

Serve with a side of mixed greens for a complete meal.

N.V.: Calories: 270, Fat: 16g, Carbs: 20g, Protein: 9g, Sugar: 4g

6. BLUEBERRY ALMOND PANCAKES

P.T.: 10 min

C.T.: 15 min

M.C.: Griddling

SERVINGS: 4

INGR.:

1 1/2 cups all-purpose flour

1/2 cup almond flour

2 tsp baking powder

1/4 tsp salt

2 Tbsp sugar

1 1/4 cups milk

1 egg

2 Tbsp melted butter

1 tsp vanilla extract

1 cup fresh blueberries

Additional butter for the pan

DIRECTIONS:

In a large bowl, whisk together all-purpose flour, almond flour, baking powder, salt, and sugar.

In another bowl, mix milk, egg, melted butter, and vanilla extract.

Pour the wet ingredients into the dry ingredients, stirring until just combined. Fold in blueberries gently.

Heat a non-stick pan or griddle over medium heat and brush with butter. Pour 1/4 cup batter for each pancake and cook until bubbles form on the surface, then flip and cook until golden brown.

TIPS:

For fluffier pancakes, let the batter rest for 5 minutes before cooking.

Serve with extra blueberries and a drizzle of maple syrup.

N.V.: Calories: 350, Fat: 15g, Carbs: 45g, Protein: 9g, Sugar: 15g

ENERGIZING LUNCHES

1. QUINOA POWER SALAD

P.T.: 15 min

C.T.: 20 min

M.C.: Boiling

SERVINGS: 4

INGR.:

1 cup quinoa

2 cups water

1/2 tsp salt

1 cup cherry tomatoes, halved

1 cucumber, diced

1/2 red onion, finely chopped

1 avocado, diced

1/4 cup fresh parsley, chopped

1/4 cup olive oil

2 Tbsp lemon juice

Salt and pepper to taste

DIRECTIONS:

Rinse quinoa under cold water. In a medium pot, bring quinoa, water, and 1/2 tsp salt to a boil. Reduce heat, cover, and simmer for 15 minutes, or until water is absorbed. Remove from heat and let sit covered for 5 minutes. Fluff with a fork.

In a large bowl, combine cooked quinoa, cherry tomatoes, cucumber, red onion, avocado, and parsley.

In a small bowl, whisk together olive oil, lemon juice, salt, and pepper. Pour dressing over salad and toss to combine.

TIPS:

Chill the salad for 1 hour before serving to enhance flavors.

Add feta cheese or chickpeas for extra protein.

N.V.: Calories: 340, Fat: 18g, Carbs: 40g, Protein: 8g, Sugar: 3g

2. SWEET POTATO LENTIL BOWL

P.T.: 10 min
C.T.: 30 min
M.C.: Roasting & Boiling
SERVINGS: 4
INGR.:

2 large sweet potatoes, peeled and cubed

1 Tbsp olive oil

Salt and pepper to taste

1 cup green lentils, rinsed

2 1/2 cups vegetable broth

1 tsp cumin

1 avocado, sliced

1/4 cup tahini

2 Tbsp lemon juice

1/4 cup water

1/4 cup fresh cilantro, chopped

DIRECTIONS:

Preheat oven to 400°F (200°C). Toss sweet potatoes with olive oil, salt, and pepper. Spread on a baking sheet and roast until tender, about 25 minutes.

In a pot, combine lentils, vegetable broth, and cumin. Bring to a boil, then simmer covered until lentils are tender, about 20 minutes.

In a small bowl, whisk together tahini, lemon juice, and water until smooth.

Divide lentils and sweet potatoes among bowls. Top with avocado slices and drizzle with tahini sauce. Garnish with cilantro.

TIPS:

Roast some red peppers alongside the sweet potatoes for added sweetness and color.

For a spicy kick, add a pinch of chili flakes to the tahini sauce.

N.V.: Calories: 450, Fat: 18g, Carbs: 62g, Protein: 15g, Sugar: 8g

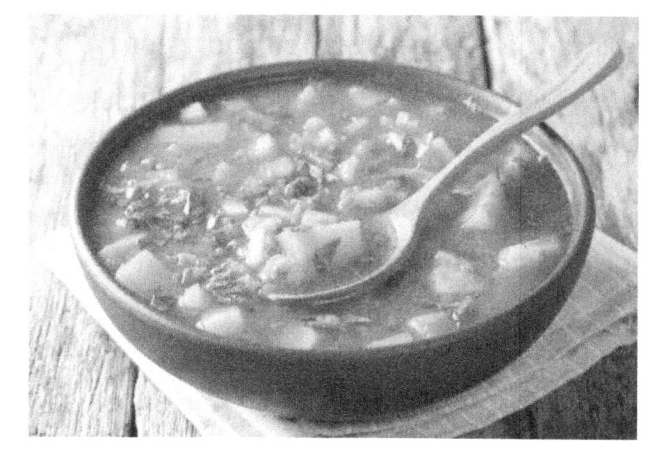

3. CHICKPEA AVOCADO WRAP

P.T.: 15 min
C.T.: 0 min
M.C.: No cook
SERVINGS: 4
INGR.:

1 can (15 oz) chickpeas, rinsed and drained
1 ripe avocado
1/4 cup Greek yogurt
1 Tbsp lemon juice
Salt and pepper to taste
1/2 cup diced cucumbers
1/2 cup diced tomatoes
1/4 cup red onion, finely chopped
4 whole wheat tortillas
1 cup mixed greens

DIRECTIONS:

In a bowl, mash the avocado and mix with chickpeas, Greek yogurt, lemon juice, salt, and pepper until well combined.

Stir in cucumbers, tomatoes, and red onion.

Lay out the tortillas and divide the chickpea mixture among them, adding a layer of mixed greens on top.

Roll up the tortillas tightly, tucking in the sides as you go.

TIPS:

For a vegan version, substitute Greek yogurt with a plant-based yogurt.

Add a sprinkle of chili flakes for a spicy twist.

N.V.: Calories: 380, Fat: 12g, Carbs: 56g, Protein: 14g, Sugar: 5g

4. TURKEY AND QUINOA STUFFED PEPPERS

P.T.: 20 min
C.T.: 35 min
M.C.: Baking
SERVINGS: 4
INGR.:

4 large bell peppers, halved and seeded
1 Tbsp olive oil
1 lb ground turkey
1 cup quinoa, cooked
1 can (15 oz) diced tomatoes, drained
1 tsp garlic powder
1 tsp onion powder
1/2 tsp smoked paprika
Salt and pepper to taste
1/2 cup shredded mozzarella cheese

DIRECTIONS:

Preheat oven to 375°F (190°C).

Place the bell pepper halves in a baking dish, cut-side up.

In a skillet, heat the olive oil over medium heat. Add the ground turkey and cook until browned.

Stir in the cooked quinoa, diced tomatoes, garlic powder, onion powder, smoked paprika, salt, and pepper. Cook for 5 more minutes.

Spoon the turkey and quinoa mixture into the bell pepper halves. Top with shredded mozzarella cheese.

Bake in the preheated oven for 25 minutes, or

until the peppers are tender and the cheese is bubbly.

TIPS:

For a vegetarian option, substitute ground turkey with additional quinoa or a plant-based meat alternative.

Serve with a side of sour cream or Greek yogurt for added creaminess.

N.V.: Calories: 420, Fat: 18g, Carbs: 38g, Protein: 32g, Sugar: 6g

5. ASIAN CHICKEN SALAD

P.T.: 20 min
C.T.: 0 min
M.C.: No cook
SERVINGS: 4
INGR.:
2 cups shredded cooked chicken
2 cups shredded cabbage
1 cup shredded carrots
1 red bell pepper, thinly sliced
1/4 cup green onions, chopped
1/4 cup cilantro, chopped
1/4 cup almonds, sliced
2 Tbsp sesame seeds

For the dressing:
1/4 cup soy sauce
2 Tbsp rice vinegar
1 Tbsp honey
1 Tbsp sesame oil
1 tsp ginger, grated
1 garlic clove, minced

DIRECTIONS:

In a large bowl, combine chicken, cabbage, carrots, bell pepper, green onions, cilantro, almonds, and sesame seeds.

In a small bowl, whisk together the dressing ingredients.

Pour the dressing over the salad and toss to coat evenly.

TIPS:

Chill the salad for 30 minutes before serving to allow flavors to meld.

Top with crispy wonton strips for extra crunch.

N.V.: Calories: 290, Fat: 14g, Carbs: 18g, Protein: 26g, Sugar: 8g

6. MEDITERRANEAN LENTIL PASTA SALAD

P.T.: 15 min
C.T.: 10 min
M.C.: Boiling
SERVINGS: 4
INGR.:
2 cups lentil pasta
1 cup cherry tomatoes, halved
1 cup cucumber, diced
1/2 cup kalamata olives, pitted and halved
1/4 cup red onion, thinly sliced
1/4 cup feta cheese, crumbled
1/4 cup parsley, chopped

For the dressing:

1/4 cup olive oil

2 Tbsp lemon juice

1 tsp dried oregano

Salt and pepper to taste

DIRECTIONS:

Cook the lentil pasta according to package instructions. Rinse under cold water and drain.

In a large bowl, combine cooked pasta, cherry tomatoes, cucumber, kalamata olives, red onion, feta cheese, and parsley.

In a small bowl, whisk together the dressing ingredients.

Pour the dressing over the pasta salad and toss to combine.

TIPS:

Add grilled chicken or shrimp for a protein boost.

Serve chilled, making it perfect for picnics or as a refreshing summer meal.

N.V.: Calories: 380, Fat: 18g, Carbs: 42g, Protein: 14g, Sugar: 4g

SATISFYING DINNERS

1. ROASTED VEGETABLE AND FARRO BOWL

P.T.: 15 min

C.T.: 30 min

M.C.: Roasting

SERVINGS: 4

INGR.:

2 cups farro, rinsed

4 cups vegetable broth

1 medium zucchini, cubed

1 red bell pepper, chopped

1 yellow bell pepper, chopped

1 red onion, sliced

2 Tbsp olive oil

Salt and pepper to taste

1/4 cup pesto

1/4 cup grated Parmesan cheese

1/4 cup toasted pine nuts

DIRECTIONS:

Preheat oven to 425°F (220°C).

In a medium saucepan, bring farro and vegetable broth to a boil. Reduce heat, cover, and simmer until farro is tender, about 30 minutes. Drain any excess liquid.

Toss zucchini, bell peppers, and red onion with olive oil, salt, and pepper on a baking sheet. Roast in the preheated oven until vegetables are tender and caramelized, about 20 minutes.

In a large bowl, combine cooked farro with roasted vegetables. Stir in pesto until evenly coated.

Serve in bowls, topped with grated Parmesan, toasted pine nuts, and additional pesto if desired.

TIPS:

Substitute any seasonal vegetables you prefer or have on hand.

For a vegan option, use a dairy-free pesto and

omit the Parmesan cheese.

N.V.: Calories: 520, Fat: 18g, Carbs: 78g, Protein: 17g, Sugar: 6g

2. LEMON HERB CHICKEN PASTA

P.T.: 20 min
C.T.: 20 min
M.C.: Boiling & Sautéing
SERVINGS: 4
INGR.:
12 oz whole wheat spaghetti
2 Tbsp olive oil
1 lb chicken breast, cut into strips
Salt and pepper to taste
1 garlic clove, minced
1 lemon, zest and juice
1/2 cup low-sodium chicken broth
1 cup cherry tomatoes, halved
1/4 cup fresh basil, chopped
1/4 cup fresh parsley, chopped
DIRECTIONS:
Cook spaghetti according to package instructions. Drain and set aside.

In a large skillet, heat 1 Tbsp olive oil over medium heat. Season chicken with salt and pepper, and sauté until golden and cooked through. Remove chicken and set aside.

In the same skillet, add remaining olive oil and garlic. Sauté for 1 minute until fragrant.

Add lemon zest, lemon juice, and chicken broth. Bring to a simmer.

Add the cooked spaghetti, cherry tomatoes, and cooked chicken back into the skillet. Toss until well combined and heated through.

Stir in basil and parsley just before serving.

TIPS:

For an extra lemony flavor, add slices of lemon when serving.

Top with grated Parmesan cheese for added richness.

N.V.: Calories: 450, Fat: 12g, Carbs: 55g, Protein: 35g, Sugar: 3g

3. BALSAMIC GLAZED SALMON WITH QUINOA AND SPINACH

P.T.: 10 min
C.T.: 20 min
M.C.: Baking & Boiling
SERVINGS: 4
INGR.:
4 salmon fillets (6 oz each)
Salt and pepper to taste
1/4 cup balsamic vinegar
2 Tbsp honey
1 cup quinoa
2 cups water
2 cups fresh spinach, roughly chopped
1 Tbsp olive oil
1 lemon, cut into wedges
DIRECTIONS:
Preheat oven to 400°F (200°C). Season salmon with salt and pepper. Place on a baking sheet lined with parchment paper.

In a small saucepan, combine balsamic vinegar and honey. Simmer over medium heat until reduced by half, about 5 minutes. Brush glaze over salmon.

Bake salmon in the preheated oven until cooked through, about 12-15 minutes.

Meanwhile, rinse quinoa under cold water. In a medium pot, bring quinoa and water to a boil. Reduce heat, cover, and simmer until water is absorbed, about 15 minutes. Stir in spinach and olive oil until spinach is wilted.

Serve salmon over a bed of quinoa and spinach, with lemon wedges on the side.

TIPS:

The balsamic glaze can also be used on chicken or roasted vegetables.

Add toasted almonds or walnuts to the quinoa for added texture and flavor.

N.V.: Calories: 500, Fat: 18g, Carbs: 45g, Protein: 42g, Sugar: 12g

4. THAI PEANUT SWEET POTATO BUDDHA BOWL

P.T.: 20 min
C.T.: 30 min
M.C.: Roasting & Boiling
SERVINGS: 4
INGR.:
2 large sweet potatoes, peeled and cubed
1 Tbsp olive oil
Salt and pepper to taste
1 cup quinoa
2 cups water
1 cup shredded red cabbage
1 cup shredded carrots
1/2 cup chopped cilantro
1/4 cup green onions, sliced
For the Thai peanut sauce:
1/4 cup peanut butter
2 Tbsp soy sauce
1 Tbsp honey
1 Tbsp lime juice
1 tsp ginger, grated
1 clove garlic, minced
Water, as needed to thin

DIRECTIONS:

Preheat oven to 425°F (220°C). Toss sweet potatoes with olive oil, salt, and pepper. Spread on a baking sheet and roast until tender, about 25 minutes.

Rinse quinoa under cold water. In a pot, bring quinoa and water to a boil, reduce heat, cover, and simmer until water is absorbed, about 15 minutes.

For the sauce, whisk together peanut butter, soy sauce, honey, lime juice, ginger, and garlic in a bowl. Add water as needed to achieve desired consistency.

Assemble the Buddha bowls by dividing quinoa, roasted sweet potatoes, red cabbage, carrots, cilantro, and green onions among four bowls. Drizzle with Thai peanut sauce before serving.

TIPS:

Garnish with chopped peanuts for extra

crunch and flavor.

Add a protein like grilled chicken or tofu to make the meal more filling.

N.V.: Calories: 520, Fat: 16g, Carbs: 82g, Protein: 14g, Sugar: 12g

---

5. MUSHROOM RISOTTO WITH PEAS

P.T.: 10 min
C.T.: 25 min
M.C.: Stirring
SERVINGS: 4
INGR.:

1 Tbsp olive oil
1 small onion, finely chopped
2 cloves garlic, minced
1 lb cremini mushrooms, sliced
1 cup Arborio rice
1/2 cup white wine
4 cups vegetable broth, warmed
1 cup frozen peas, thawed
1/2 cup Parmesan cheese, grated
Salt and pepper to taste
Fresh parsley, chopped for garnish

DIRECTIONS:

In a large pan, heat olive oil over medium heat. Add onion and garlic, sautéing until softened.

Add mushrooms and cook until they release their moisture and begin to brown.

Stir in Arborio rice, coating it in the oil. Pour in white wine and stir until absorbed.

Gradually add warm vegetable broth, one ladle at a time, stirring constantly. Wait until each addition is almost fully absorbed before adding the next.

When the rice is creamy and just tender, stir in peas, Parmesan cheese, salt, and pepper. Cook until peas are heated through.

Serve garnished with fresh parsley.

TIPS:

For a vegan version, omit the Parmesan or use a plant-based alternative.

Toasting the rice before adding liquids enhances the risotto's nutty flavor.

N.V.: Calories: 420, Fat: 12g, Carbs: 62g, Protein: 15g, Sugar: 5g

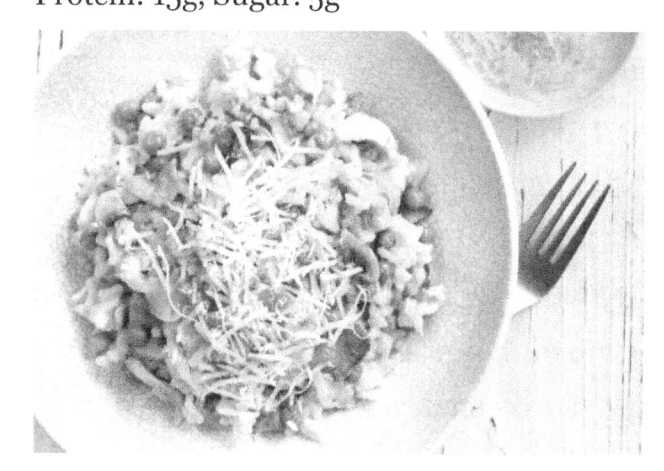

---

6. CREAMY COCONUT LENTIL CURRY

P.T.: 15 min
C.T.: 20 min
M.C.: Simmering
SERVINGS: 4
INGR.:
1 Tbsp coconut oil

1 onion, diced

2 cloves garlic, minced

1 Tbsp curry powder

1 tsp ground turmeric

1 tsp ground cumin

1 can (14 oz) coconut milk

1 can (14 oz) diced tomatoes

1 cup red lentils

3 cups spinach leaves

Salt and pepper to taste

Cooked rice, for serving

Fresh cilantro, for garnish

DIRECTIONS:

In a large pot, heat coconut oil over medium heat. Add onion and garlic, cooking until the onion is translucent.

Stir in curry powder, turmeric, and cumin, cooking until fragrant.

Add coconut milk, diced tomatoes (with juices), and red lentils. Bring to a simmer and cook, uncovered, stirring occasionally, until lentils are tender, about 20 minutes.

Stir in spinach until wilted. Season with salt and pepper to taste.

Serve over cooked rice, garnished with fresh cilantro.

TIPS:

Squeeze fresh lime juice over the curry before serving for added brightness.

Add chili pepper flakes while cooking if you prefer a spicier curry.

N.V.: Calories: 480, Fat: 22g, Carbs: 58g, Protein: 18g, Sugar: 6g

SNACKS AND SMOOTHIES

1. TROPICAL GREEN SMOOTHIE

P.T.: 5 min

C.T.: 0 min

M.C.: Blending

SERVINGS: 2

INGR.:

1 cup fresh spinach

1/2 cup coconut water

1 banana, sliced and frozen

1/2 cup mango chunks, frozen

1/2 cup pineapple chunks, frozen

1 Tbsp chia seeds

DIRECTIONS:

In a blender, combine spinach and coconut water. Blend until smooth.

Add the frozen banana, mango, and pineapple chunks. Blend again until smooth and creamy.

Stir in chia seeds after blending.

TIPS:

For an extra boost, add a scoop of your favorite protein powder.

If the smoothie is too thick, add more coconut water until desired consistency is reached.

N.V.: Calories: 180, Fat: 2g, Carbs: 42g, Protein: 3g, Sugar: 28g

2. PEANUT BUTTER ENERGY BALLS

P.T.: 10 min
C.T.: 0 min
M.C.: No cook
SERVINGS: 12 balls
INGR.:

1 cup rolled oats

1/2 cup natural peanut butter

1/3 cup honey

1/4 cup ground flaxseed

1/2 cup mini chocolate chips

1 tsp vanilla extract

DIRECTIONS:

In a medium bowl, mix together the rolled oats, peanut butter, honey, ground flaxseed, mini chocolate chips, and vanilla extract until well combined.

Roll the mixture into balls, about 1 inch in diameter.

Place the energy balls on a baking sheet lined with parchment paper and refrigerate for at least 30 minutes before serving.

TIPS:

Store in an airtight container in the refrigerator for up to a week.

Substitute almond butter or cashew butter for a different flavor.

N.V.: Calories: 150, Fat: 8g, Carbs: 18g, Protein: 4g, Sugar: 12g

3. AVOCADO TOAST WITH TOMATO AND BASIL

P.T.: 5 min
C.T.: 0 min
M.C.: Toasting
SERVINGS: 2
INGR.:

2 slices whole grain bread

1 ripe avocado

Salt and pepper to taste

1/2 cup cherry tomatoes, halved

Fresh basil leaves

Balsamic glaze (optional)

DIRECTIONS:

Toast the whole grain bread to your liking.

Mash the avocado in a bowl with a fork. Season with salt and pepper.

Spread the mashed avocado evenly on the toasted bread.

Top with halved cherry tomatoes and fresh basil leaves.

Drizzle with balsamic glaze if desired.

TIPS:

For added protein, top with a poached or fried egg.

Sprinkle with red pepper flakes for a spicy kick.

N.V.: Calories: 250, Fat: 14g, Carbs: 27g, Protein: 6g, Sugar: 4g

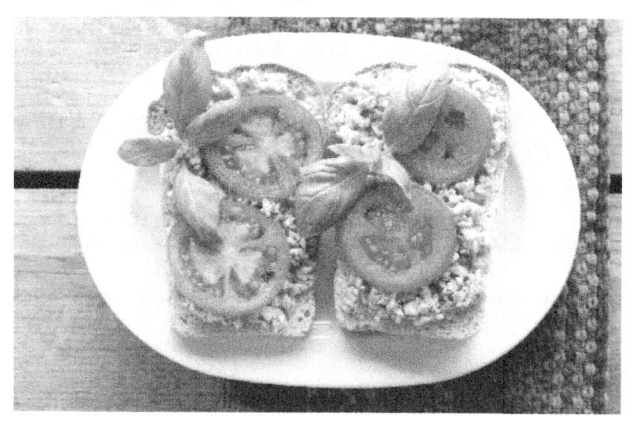

4. CINNAMON APPLE CHIPS

P.T.: 10 min
C.T.: 2 hr
M.C.: Baking
SERVINGS: 4
INGR.:
2 large apples
1 tsp ground cinnamon
1 Tbsp sugar (optional)
DIRECTIONS:
Preheat oven to 200°F (93°C). Line two baking sheets with parchment paper.
Core the apples and slice them very thinly.
Arrange apple slices in a single layer on the baking sheets.
Mix cinnamon and sugar together and sprinkle over the apple slices.
Bake for 1 hour, flip the slices, then bake for another 1 hour until the apple slices are crisp.
Let cool completely before serving.
TIPS:
For extra crispiness, let the apple chips cool in the oven after turning it off.
Experiment with different apple varieties for a range of flavors and sweetness.
N.V.: Calories: 50, Fat: 0g, Carbs: 13g, Protein: 0g, Sugar: 10g

5. BERRY BANANA SMOOTHIE BOWL

P.T.: 10 min
C.T.: 0 min
M.C.: Blending
SERVINGS: 2
INGR.:
1 frozen banana
1/2 cup frozen mixed berries
1/2 cup Greek yogurt
1/4 cup almond milk
1 Tbsp honey
Toppings: sliced fresh fruit, granola, chia seeds, shredded coconut
DIRECTIONS:
In a blender, combine the frozen banana, mixed berries, Greek yogurt, almond milk, and honey. Blend until smooth.
Pour the smoothie mixture into bowls.
Top with your choice of sliced fresh fruit, granola, chia seeds, and shredded coconut.
TIPS:
Adjust the thickness by adding more or less almond milk.
For added protein, mix in a scoop of your favorite protein powder.
N.V.: Calories: 220, Fat: 2g, Carbs: 44g, Protein: 8g, Sugar: 30g

6. HUMMUS AND VEGGIE ROLL-UPS

P.T.: 15 min
C.T.: 0 min
M.C.: No cook
SERVINGS: 4

INGR.:

4 whole wheat tortillas

1 cup hummus

1 carrot, julienned

1 cucumber, julienned

1 red bell pepper, julienned

1 avocado, sliced

1/4 cup spinach leaves

Salt and pepper to taste

DIRECTIONS:

Lay out the tortillas on a flat surface. Spread each tortilla with a layer of hummus.

Distribute the julienned vegetables and avocado slices evenly among the tortillas. Add a few spinach leaves to each.

Season with salt and pepper.

Roll up the tortillas tightly, then cut into pieces if desired.

TIPS:

For a gluten-free option, use corn tortillas instead of whole wheat.

Add a sprinkle of chili flakes or a drizzle of tahini for extra flavor.

N.V.: Calories: 320, Fat: 15g, Carbs: 40g, Protein: 10g, Sugar: 5g

CHAPTER 4: LOW-CARB DAY RECIPES

MORNING STARTERS

1. SPINACH AND FETA OMELETTE

P.T.: 5 min
C.T.: 10 min
M.C.: Sautéing & Flipping
SERVINGS: 2
INGR.:
4 large eggs
2 Tbsp water
Salt and pepper to taste
1 Tbsp olive oil
1 cup fresh spinach, chopped
1/2 cup feta cheese, crumbled
1/4 cup red onion, diced

DIRECTIONS:
In a bowl, whisk together eggs, water, salt, and pepper.
Heat olive oil in a non-stick skillet over medium heat. Sauté red onion until translucent, about 3 minutes.
Add spinach to the skillet and cook until just wilted.
Pour the egg mixture over the spinach and onions. Cook until the eggs begin to set on the bottom.
Sprinkle feta cheese over one half of the omelette. Fold the other half over the cheese.
Cook for another 2 minutes, then flip carefully and cook for 2 more minutes or until the eggs are fully set.

TIPS:
For a fluffy omelette, add a splash of milk to the eggs.
Serve with a side of avocado slices for added healthy fats.

N.V.: Calories: 320, Fat: 24g, Carbs: 4g, Protein: 20g, Sugar: 2g

2. ALMOND FLOUR PANCAKES

P.T.: 10 min
C.T.: 15 min
M.C.: Griddling
SERVINGS: 4
INGR.:
1 1/2 cups almond flour
3 large eggs
1/2 cup almond milk
1 Tbsp coconut oil, melted
1 tsp baking powder
1/4 tsp salt
1 tsp vanilla extract
Sugar-free maple syrup, for serving

DIRECTIONS:
In a large bowl, combine almond flour, eggs, almond milk, melted coconut oil, baking powder, salt, and vanilla extract. Stir until well combined.
Heat a non-stick skillet or griddle over medium heat. Pour 1/4 cup of batter for each

pancake. Cook until bubbles form on the surface, then flip and cook until golden brown on the other side.

Serve hot with sugar-free maple syrup.

TIPS:

If the batter is too thick, add more almond milk to reach desired consistency.

Add blueberries or chocolate chips to the batter for added flavor.

N.V.: Calories: 280, Fat: 23g, Carbs: 8g, Protein: 12g, Sugar: 2g

3. AVOCADO AND EGG BREAKFAST BOWL

P.T.: 5 min
C.T.: 10 min
M.C.: Boiling & Assembling
SERVINGS: 2
INGR.:
4 eggs
1 avocado, halved and sliced
2 cups spinach leaves
1/4 cup cherry tomatoes, halved
1/4 tsp chili flakes
Salt and pepper to taste
1 Tbsp olive oil
DIRECTIONS:

Boil eggs to your preferred level of doneness.

In a bowl, arrange a bed of spinach leaves.

Top with sliced avocado, halved cherry tomatoes, and peeled, halved eggs.

Season with chili flakes, salt, and pepper.

Drizzle with olive oil before serving.

TIPS:

For added crunch, sprinkle with seeds or nuts of your choice.

A dash of lemon juice over the avocado can add a refreshing tang and prevent browning.

N.V.: Calories: 330, Fat: 27g, Carbs: 8g, Protein: 15g, Sugar: 2g

4. COTTAGE CHEESE AND BERRY PARFAIT

P.T.: 5 min
C.T.: 0 min
M.C.: Layering
SERVINGS: 2
INGR.:
1 cup cottage cheese
1/2 cup mixed berries (strawberries, blueberries, raspberries)
1 Tbsp almonds, sliced
1 Tbsp chia seeds
1 tsp honey (optional)

DIRECTIONS:

In serving glasses or bowls, layer half of the cottage cheese, followed by a layer of mixed berries.

Sprinkle half of the almonds and chia seeds over the berries.

Repeat the layers with the remaining ingredients.

Drizzle with honey if desired.

TIPS:

For a dairy-free option, use almond or

coconut yogurt in place of cottage cheese. Freeze the berries beforehand for a chilled parfait.

N.V.: Calories: 200, Fat: 8g, Carbs: 14g, Protein: 18g, Sugar: 8g

5. SMOKED SALMON AND CREAM CHEESE ROLL-UPS

P.T.: 10 min
C.T.: 0 min
M.C.: Rolling
SERVINGS: 4
INGR.:
4 oz smoked salmon, thinly sliced
4 Tbsp cream cheese, softened
1/2 cucumber, thinly sliced
1 Tbsp dill, chopped
1 tsp lemon zest
Pepper to taste
DIRECTIONS:
Lay out slices of smoked salmon on a flat surface.
Spread a thin layer of cream cheese over each slice of salmon.
Arrange cucumber slices over the cream cheese. Sprinkle with dill, lemon zest, and pepper.
Carefully roll up the salmon slices tightly. Slice into bite-sized pieces if desired.
TIPS:
Serve with lemon wedges for added zest.
Capers can be added for an extra burst of flavor.
N.V.: Calories: 120, Fat: 8g, Carbs: 2g, Protein: 10g, Sugar: 1g

6. KETO AVOCADO CHOCOLATE SMOOTHIE

P.T.: 5 min
C.T.: 0 min
M.C.: Blending
SERVINGS: 2
INGR.:
1 ripe avocado
1 cup almond milk
2 Tbsp cocoa powder
1 Tbsp almond butter
1 tsp vanilla extract
Sweetener to taste (erythritol, stevia, or monk fruit)
Ice cubes
DIRECTIONS:
Combine all ingredients in a blender.
Blend until smooth and creamy. Adjust sweetener to taste.
Serve immediately, garnished with a sprinkle of cocoa powder or sliced almonds if desired.
TIPS:
For a protein boost, add a scoop of your favorite low-carb protein powder.
Ensure the smoothie is well blended to avoid chunks of avocado.
N.V.: Calories: 250, Fat: 20g, Carbs: 12g (Net Carbs: 4g), Protein: 5g, Sugar: 1g

LIGHT AND FRESH LUNCHES

1. GRILLED CHICKEN AND AVOCADO SALAD

P.T.: 15 min
C.T.: 10 min
M.C.: Grilling
SERVINGS: 4
INGR.:
4 boneless, skinless chicken breasts
Salt and pepper to taste
2 Tbsp olive oil
2 avocados, diced
1 cup cherry tomatoes, halved
1/4 cup red onion, thinly sliced
2 Tbsp fresh lime juice
1/4 cup cilantro, chopped
1 jalapeño, seeded and minced (optional)
DIRECTIONS:
Preheat the grill to medium-high heat. Season chicken breasts with salt, pepper, and 1 Tbsp olive oil.
Grill the chicken for 5 minutes on each side or until fully cooked. Let it rest for 5 minutes, then slice.
In a large bowl, combine diced avocado, cherry tomatoes, red onion, lime juice, remaining olive oil, cilantro, and jalapeño. Add salt and pepper to taste.
Add the sliced chicken to the salad and gently toss to combine.
TIPS:
For a zestier flavor, add more lime juice or zest to the salad.
Serve over a bed of mixed greens for an even fresher approach.
N.V.: Calories: 350, Fat: 20g, Carbs: 8g, Protein: 35g, Sugar: 2g

2. ZUCCHINI NOODLE CAPRESE

P.T.: 10 min
C.T.: 0 min
M.C.: Spiralizing
SERVINGS: 2
INGR.:
2 medium zucchinis
1 cup cherry tomatoes, halved
4 oz mozzarella balls, halved
2 Tbsp pesto
1 Tbsp balsamic glaze
Salt and pepper to taste
Fresh basil leaves for garnish
DIRECTIONS:
Use a spiralizer to turn the zucchinis into noodles. Place them in a large bowl.
Add the cherry tomatoes, mozzarella balls, and pesto to the zucchini noodles. Toss to coat evenly.
Drizzle with balsamic glaze and season with salt and pepper.
Garnish with fresh basil leaves before serving.
TIPS:
For added protein, top with grilled chicken or shrimp.

Let the salad sit for 10 minutes before serving to allow the flavors to meld.

N.V.: Calories: 280, Fat: 18g, Carbs: 10g, Protein: 18g, Sugar: 6g

3. CUCUMBER SHRIMP AVOCADO SALAD

P.T.: 15 min
C.T.: 0 min
M.C.: Mixing
SERVINGS: 4
INGR.:
1 lb cooked shrimp, peeled and deveined
2 avocados, diced
2 cucumbers, diced
1/4 cup red onion, finely chopped
2 Tbsp fresh lime juice
2 Tbsp olive oil
Salt and pepper to taste
1/4 cup fresh cilantro, chopped
DIRECTIONS:

In a large bowl, combine shrimp, avocados, cucumbers, and red onion.

In a small bowl, whisk together lime juice, olive oil, salt, and pepper.

Pour the dressing over the shrimp mixture and toss gently to coat.

Garnish with chopped cilantro before serving.

TIPS:

Chill the salad for 30 minutes before serving for a refreshing touch.

For a spicy version, add diced jalapeño or chili flakes.

N.V.: Calories: 290, Fat: 18g, Carbs: 8g, Protein: 25g, Sugar: 2g

4. CAULIFLOWER RICE STIR-FRY WITH VEGETABLES

P.T.: 10 min
C.T.: 15 min
M.C.: Stir-frying
SERVINGS: 4
INGR.:
1 head cauliflower, grated into 'rice'
2 Tbsp coconut oil
1 red bell pepper, diced
1 cup snap peas, sliced
1 carrot, julienned
2 garlic cloves, minced
1 Tbsp ginger, minced
2 Tbsp soy sauce or tamari
2 eggs, beaten (optional)
Salt and pepper to taste
Green onions and sesame seeds for garnish
DIRECTIONS:

Heat coconut oil in a large skillet over medium heat. Add garlic and ginger, sautéing until fragrant, about 1 minute.

Increase heat to medium-high and add the red bell pepper, snap peas, and carrot. Stir-fry for about 5 minutes, or until vegetables are tender-crisp.

Add the cauliflower rice and soy sauce. Stir well to combine and cook for another 5-7 minutes, or until the cauliflower is tender. Make a well in the center of the skillet, add the beaten eggs, and scramble until fully cooked, then mix into the cauliflower rice. Season with salt and pepper, garnish with green onions and sesame seeds before serving.

TIPS:

For added protein, include chicken, shrimp, or tofu.

Customize with any vegetables you have on hand for a versatile meal.

N.V.: Calories: 180, Fat: 10g, Carbs: 15g, Protein: 8g, Sugar: 5g

5. GREEK CHICKEN SALAD

P.T.: 20 min
C.T.: 0 min
M.C.: Mixing
SERVINGS: 4
INGR.:
2 cups cooked chicken, shredded
1 cucumber, diced
1 cup cherry tomatoes, halved
1/2 red onion, thinly sliced
1/2 cup Kalamata olives, pitted
1/2 cup feta cheese, crumbled
2 Tbsp olive oil
1 Tbsp red wine vinegar
1 tsp dried oregano
Salt and pepper to taste
Romaine lettuce leaves for serving
DIRECTIONS:

In a large bowl, combine shredded chicken, cucumber, cherry tomatoes, red onion, Kalamata olives, and feta cheese.

In a small bowl, whisk together olive oil, red wine vinegar, dried oregano, salt, and pepper to create the dressing.

Pour the dressing over the salad and toss to coat evenly.

Serve the salad on a bed of romaine lettuce leaves.

TIPS:

Add avocado slices for extra creaminess and healthy fats.

For a zestier flavor, squeeze fresh lemon juice over the salad before serving.

N.V.: Calories: 280, Fat: 18g, Carbs: 6g, Protein: 24g, Sugar: 3g

6. BROCCOLI AND CHEESE STUFFED PEPPERS

P.T.: 15 min
C.T.: 25 min
M.C.: Baking
SERVINGS: 4
INGR.:
4 large bell peppers, halved and seeded
2 cups broccoli florets, finely chopped
1 cup cottage cheese
1/2 cup shredded cheddar cheese
1/4 cup Parmesan cheese, grated
1 garlic clove, minced
Salt and pepper to taste

1/2 tsp smoked paprika

DIRECTIONS:

Preheat oven to 375°F (190°C). Place the bell pepper halves in a baking dish, cut-side up.

In a bowl, mix together broccoli, cottage cheese, half of the cheddar cheese, Parmesan cheese, garlic, salt, pepper, and smoked paprika.

Spoon the mixture evenly into the bell pepper halves. Sprinkle with the remaining cheddar cheese.

Cover with foil and bake for 20 minutes. Remove the foil and bake for an additional 5 minutes, or until the cheese is bubbly and golden.

TIPS:

For a meaty version, add cooked ground turkey or chicken to the filling.

Serve with a side of mixed greens for a complete meal.

N.V.: Calories: 220, Fat: 12g, Carbs: 12g, Protein: 16g, Sugar: 5g

HEARTY DINNERS

1. HERB-CRUSTED SALMON WITH ASPARAGUS

P.T.: 10 min
C.T.: 20 min
M.C.: Baking
SERVINGS: 4
INGR.:
4 salmon fillets (6 oz each)
1 lb asparagus, ends trimmed
2 Tbsp olive oil
Salt and pepper to taste
For the herb crust:
1/4 cup fresh parsley, finely chopped
1/4 cup fresh dill, finely chopped
2 cloves garlic, minced
Zest of 1 lemon
2 Tbsp almond flour

DIRECTIONS:

Preheat oven to 400°F (200°C). Line a baking sheet with parchment paper.

Place salmon fillets and asparagus on the baking sheet. Drizzle with olive oil and season with salt and pepper.

In a small bowl, mix together parsley, dill, garlic, lemon zest, and almond flour. Press the herb mixture onto the top of each salmon fillet.

Bake for 15-20 minutes, or until the salmon is cooked through and the asparagus is tender.

TIPS:

Ensure not to overcook the salmon; it should be moist and flaky.

Squeeze fresh lemon juice over the cooked salmon and asparagus for added zest.

N.V.: Calories: 300, Fat: 18g, Carbs: 6g, Protein: 29g, Sugar: 2g

2. BEEF AND BROCCOLI STIR-FRY

P.T.: 15 min
C.T.: 10 min
M.C.: Stir-frying
SERVINGS: 4
INGR.:

1 lb flank steak, thinly sliced
1 Tbsp sesame oil
4 cups broccoli florets
1/4 cup soy sauce
2 cloves garlic, minced
1 Tbsp ginger, grated
1 tsp erythritol or other sugar substitute
2 tsp apple cider vinegar
Salt and pepper to taste
Sesame seeds for garnish

DIRECTIONS:

Heat sesame oil in a large skillet over medium-high heat. Add the flank steak and stir-fry until browned and cooked to your liking. Remove from skillet and set aside.

In the same skillet, add broccoli florets and stir-fry until tender but still crisp.

Add the soy sauce, garlic, ginger, erythritol, and apple cider vinegar to the skillet. Return the beef to the skillet and toss to combine with the broccoli and sauce.

Season with salt and pepper to taste. Garnish with sesame seeds before serving.

TIPS:

For a thicker sauce, add a slurry of 1 tsp arrowroot powder mixed with 2 tsp water.

Serve over cauliflower rice for a complete low-carb meal.

N.V.: Calories: 280, Fat: 14g, Carbs: 8g, Protein: 30g, Sugar: 3g

3. GRILLED PORK CHOPS WITH HERB BUTTER

P.T.: 10 min (plus marinating time)
C.T.: 12 min
M.C.: Grilling
SERVINGS: 4
INGR.:

4 pork chops, bone-in, 1-inch thick
2 Tbsp olive oil
Salt and pepper to taste
For the herb butter:
4 Tbsp unsalted butter, softened
1 Tbsp fresh rosemary, chopped
1 Tbsp fresh thyme, chopped
2 cloves garlic, minced
Zest of 1 lemon

DIRECTIONS:

Season pork chops with olive oil, salt, and pepper. Let marinate for at least 30 minutes.

Preheat grill to medium-high heat. Grill pork chops for 5-6 minutes on each side or until the internal temperature reaches 145°F (63°C).

Meanwhile, in a small bowl, mix together the butter, rosemary, thyme, garlic, and lemon zest.

Top each grilled pork chop with a dollop of herb butter before serving.

TIPS:

Let the pork chops rest for 5 minutes after grilling to retain their juices.

The herb butter can also be used on vegetables or other meats.

N.V.: Calories: 350, Fat: 25g, Carbs: 1g, Protein: 30g, Sugar: 0g

4. CAJUN SHRIMP AND AVOCADO SALAD

P.T.: 10 min
C.T.: 5 min
M.C.: Sautéing
SERVINGS: 4
INGR.:

1 lb large shrimp, peeled and deveined

2 Tbsp Cajun seasoning

1 Tbsp olive oil

2 avocados, diced

1 cup cherry tomatoes, halved

1/4 cup red onion, thinly sliced

2 Tbsp fresh lime juice

Salt and pepper to taste

Mixed greens for serving

DIRECTIONS:

Toss shrimp with Cajun seasoning until evenly coated.

Heat olive oil in a skillet over medium-high heat. Add the shrimp and sauté for 2-3 minutes on each side, or until fully cooked and slightly charred.

In a large bowl, combine diced avocados, cherry tomatoes, and red onion. Add the cooked shrimp. Drizzle with lime juice and season with salt and pepper. Toss gently to combine.

Serve the salad over a bed of mixed greens.

TIPS:

Adjust the amount of Cajun seasoning to suit your spice preference.

Add cucumber or bell pepper for extra crunch and freshness.

N.V.: Calories: 290, Fat: 18g, Carbs: 9g, Protein: 25g, Sugar: 2g

5. TURKEY BACON WRAPPED ASPARAGUS

P.T.: 10 min
C.T.: 15 min
M.C.: Baking
SERVINGS: 4
INGR.:

16 asparagus spears, trimmed

8 slices turkey bacon

1 Tbsp olive oil

Salt and pepper to taste

DIRECTIONS:

Preheat oven to 400°F (200°C). Line a baking sheet with parchment paper.

Wrap each asparagus spear with half a slice of turkey bacon. Arrange on the prepared baking sheet.

Lightly brush the asparagus and bacon with olive oil. Season with salt and pepper.

Bake for 15 minutes, or until the bacon is

crispy and the asparagus is tender.

TIPS:

For a smokey flavor, sprinkle a little paprika on top before baking.

Serve with a side of low-carb aioli or mustard for dipping.

N.V.: Calories: 120, Fat: 7g, Carbs: 3g, Protein: 10g, Sugar: 1g

6. SPICY KALE AND CHICKEN SOUP

P.T.: 15 min
C.T.: 30 min
M.C.: Simmering
SERVINGS: 6
INGR.:
1 Tbsp olive oil
1 lb chicken breast, diced
1 onion, diced
2 garlic cloves, minced
1 tsp chili flakes (adjust to taste)
6 cups chicken broth
4 cups kale, stemmed and chopped
Salt and pepper to taste
Juice of 1 lemon

DIRECTIONS:

Heat olive oil in a large pot over medium heat. Add diced chicken and cook until browned. Remove chicken and set aside.

In the same pot, add onion and garlic. Sauté until softened.

Add chili flakes, chicken broth, and cooked chicken. Bring to a simmer.

Add chopped kale and simmer for another 15-20 minutes, or until the kale is tender and the chicken is fully cooked.

Season with salt and pepper to taste. Stir in lemon juice just before serving.

TIPS:

Substitute kale with spinach or Swiss chard if preferred.

Add low-carb vegetables like zucchini or bell peppers for more variety.

N.V.: Calories: 180, Fat: 5g, Carbs: 6g, Protein: 27g, Sugar: 2g

LOW-CARB SNACKS AND TREATS

1. CHEESY KALE CHIPS

P.T.: 10 min
C.T.: 20 min
M.C.: Baking
SERVINGS: 4
INGR.:
1 bunch kale, stems removed and leaves torn
1 Tbsp olive oil
1/4 cup grated Parmesan cheese
Salt to taste

DIRECTIONS:

Preheat oven to 300°F (150°C). Line a baking sheet with parchment paper.

In a large bowl, toss kale leaves with olive oil and salt until evenly coated.

Arrange kale on the baking sheet in a single layer. Sprinkle with grated Parmesan cheese. Bake for 20 minutes or until the edges are crisp but not browned. Let cool before serving.
TIPS:

Ensure kale leaves are dry before tossing with oil for the crispiest chips.

Store in an airtight container to keep them crispy for longer.

N.V.: Calories: 80, Fat: 5g, Carbs: 5g, Protein: 4g, Sugar: 0g

2. AVOCADO DEVILED EGGS

P.T.: 15 min
C.T.: 0 min
M.C.: Mixing
SERVINGS: 6 (12 halves)
INGR.:
6 hard-boiled eggs, peeled
1 ripe avocado
1 Tbsp lime juice
Salt and pepper to taste
Paprika for garnish
Chopped cilantro for garnish
DIRECTIONS:
Halve the eggs lengthwise. Remove yolks and place in a bowl.

Mash the yolks with avocado and lime juice. Season with salt and pepper.

Spoon or pipe the mixture back into the egg whites.

Sprinkle with paprika and garnish with chopped cilantro before serving.

TIPS:

For a smoother filling, use a food processor to blend the yolks and avocado.

Add a dash of hot sauce to the filling for an extra kick.

N.V.: Calories: 100, Fat: 8g, Carbs: 2g, Protein: 6g, Sugar: 1g

3. CUCUMBER TUNA BOATS

P.T.: 10 min
C.T.: 0 min
M.C.: Assembling
SERVINGS: 4
INGR.:
2 large cucumbers, halved and seeds removed
1 can (5 oz) tuna in water, drained
1/4 cup mayonnaise
1 Tbsp Dijon mustard
1/4 cup red onion, finely diced

Salt and pepper to taste
Fresh dill for garnish
DIRECTIONS:
In a bowl, mix together tuna, mayonnaise, Dijon mustard, and red onion. Season with salt and pepper.

Spoon the tuna mixture into the hollowed-out cucumber halves.

Garnish with fresh dill before serving.

TIPS:

For added crunch, mix in some chopped celery or bell pepper to the tuna mixture.

Serve chilled for a refreshing snack or light lunch.

N.V.: Calories: 150, Fat: 10g, Carbs: 4g, Protein: 12g, Sugar: 2g

4. BAKED PEPPERONI CHIPS

P.T.: 5 min
C.T.: 10 min
M.C.: Baking
SERVINGS: 4
INGR.:

4 oz pepperoni slices

DIRECTIONS:

Preheat oven to 400°F (200°C). Line a baking sheet with parchment paper.

Arrange pepperoni slices in a single layer on the baking sheet.

Bake for 8-10 minutes or until crisp.

Transfer to a paper towel-lined plate to absorb any excess grease. Let cool before serving.

TIPS:

Watch the pepperoni closely as it can go from crisp to burnt quickly.

Pair with a side of low-carb marinara sauce for dipping.

N.V.: Calories: 140, Fat: 12g, Carbs: 0g, Protein: 8g, Sugar: 0g

5. ALMOND BUTTER CELERY STICKS

P.T.: 5 min
C.T.: 0 min
M.C.: Assembling
SERVINGS: 4
INGR.:

8 celery stalks, trimmed and cleaned
1/2 cup almond butter
1/4 cup raisins (optional)

DIRECTIONS:

Fill each celery stalk with almond butter.

Sprinkle raisins on top of the almond butter, if using.

Serve immediately or chill in the refrigerator before serving for a refreshing snack.

TIPS:

For added texture and flavor, sprinkle with a little sea salt or drizzle with honey.

Substitute raisins with dried cranberries or chopped nuts for variety.

N.V.: Calories: 200, Fat: 16g, Carbs: 8g (subtract 2g if omitting raisins), Protein: 6g, Sugar: 4g

6. MINI BELL PEPPER NACHOS

P.T.: 10 min

C.T.: 15 min

M.C.: Baking

SERVINGS: 4

INGR.:

12 mini bell peppers, halved and seeds removed

1 cup cooked ground turkey, seasoned with taco seasoning

1/2 cup shredded cheddar cheese

1/4 cup black olives, sliced

1/4 cup green onions, chopped

Sour cream and salsa for serving

DIRECTIONS:

Preheat oven to 375°F (190°C). Arrange bell pepper halves on a baking sheet.

Spoon the cooked, seasoned ground turkey into each bell pepper half.

Sprinkle with shredded cheddar cheese.

Bake for 10-15 minutes or until the cheese is melted and bubbly.

Garnish with sliced black olives and chopped green onions. Serve with sour cream and salsa on the side.

TIPS:

For a vegetarian version, substitute ground turkey with a mix of black beans and corn.

Add a drizzle of guacamole or diced avocado on top for extra creaminess and flavor.

N.V.: Calories: 220, Fat: 12g, Carbs: 8g, Protein: 20g, Sugar: 4g

CHAPTER 5: BALANCED MEALS FOR TRANSITION DAYS

NUTRIENT-RICH BREAKFASTS

1. SUNRISE TURMERIC QUINOA BOWL

P.T.: 10 min
C.T.: 20 min
M.C.: Simmering
SERVINGS: 4
INGR.:
1 cup quinoa, rinsed
2 cups water
1 tsp turmeric
1/2 tsp cinnamon
1/4 tsp salt
1 apple, diced
1/4 cup raisins
1/4 cup walnuts, chopped
1/4 cup unsweetened almond milk
2 Tblsp maple syrup
DIRECTIONS:

In a saucepan, combine quinoa, water, turmeric, cinnamon, and salt. Bring to a boil, then cover and simmer for 15 minutes or until water is absorbed.

Stir in diced apple, raisins, and walnuts. Cook for an additional 5 minutes.

Divide into bowls and drizzle with almond milk and maple syrup before serving.

TIPS:

Top with a dollop of Greek yogurt for added protein.

Sprinkle with chia seeds for an omega-3 boost.

N.V.: Calories: 320, Fat: 9g, Carbs: 52g, Protein: 8g, Sugar: 15g

2. GREEN GODDESS AVOCADO TOAST

P.T.: 5 min
C.T.: 0 min
M.C.: Toasting
SERVINGS: 2
INGR.:
4 slices whole grain bread, toasted
2 ripe avocados, mashed
1/2 cup baby spinach, finely chopped
1/4 cup feta cheese, crumbled
2 tsp lemon juice
Salt and pepper to taste
Red pepper flakes (optional)

DIRECTIONS:

In a bowl, mix mashed avocados, spinach, lemon juice, salt, and pepper.

Spread the mixture evenly on toasted bread slices.

Top with crumbled feta and red pepper flakes if desired.

TIPS:

For a protein-rich breakfast, add a poached egg on top.

Drizzle with a bit of olive oil for extra richness.

N.V.: Calories: 370, Fat: 22g, Carbs: 35g, Protein: 9g, Sugar: 5g

3. BERRY CHIA OVERNIGHT OATS

P.T.: 10 min (overnight soaking)
C.T.: 0 min
M.C.: Refrigeration
SERVINGS: 4
INGR.:
2 cups rolled oats
4 Tblsp chia seeds
2 cups unsweetened almond milk
1 cup mixed berries (fresh or frozen)
1 Tblsp honey (optional)
1 tsp vanilla extract
DIRECTIONS:

In a large bowl, mix oats, chia seeds, almond milk, honey, and vanilla extract.

Stir in half of the berries.

Cover and refrigerate overnight.

Serve topped with the remaining berries.

TIPS:

Add a scoop of protein powder for an extra protein kick.

Substitute almond milk with any milk of your choice.

N.V.: Calories: 290, Fat: 8g, Carbs: 46g, Protein: 10g, Sugar: 8g

4. SAVORY MUSHROOM AND SPINACH FRITTATA

P.T.: 15 min
C.T.: 25 min
M.C.: Baking
SERVINGS: 4
INGR.:
8 eggs
1/2 cup milk
1 cup mushrooms, sliced
2 cups spinach, roughly chopped
1/2 cup grated Parmesan cheese
1/4 tsp salt
1/4 tsp black pepper
1 Tblsp olive oil
DIRECTIONS:
Preheat oven to 375°F (190°C).
In a skillet, heat olive oil over medium heat.

Add mushrooms and sauté until tender. Add spinach and cook until wilted.

In a bowl, whisk eggs, milk, salt, and pepper.

Stir in cooked mushrooms, spinach, and half of the Parmesan cheese.

Pour the mixture into a greased baking dish.

Sprinkle with the remaining Parmesan cheese. Bake for 25 minutes or until the frittata is set and golden.

TIPS:

Serve with a side of mixed greens for a complete meal.

For a fluffier frittata, use half-and-half instead of milk.

N.V.: Calories: 300, Fat: 20g, Carbs: 6g, Protein: 24g, Sugar: 3g

5. SMOKED SALMON BREAKFAST SALAD

P.T.: 10 min
C.T.: 0 min
M.C.: Assembly
SERVINGS: 2
INGR.:
4 cups mixed salad greens
4 oz smoked salmon, thinly sliced
2 hard-boiled eggs, quartered
1 avocado, sliced
2 Tblsp capers
Dressing: 2 Tblsp olive oil, 1 Tblsp lemon juice, salt, and pepper
DIRECTIONS:
Arrange salad greens on plates.
Top with smoked salmon, eggs, avocado slices, and capers.
Whisk together olive oil, lemon juice, salt, and pepper. Drizzle over the salad.
TIPS:
Add a sprinkle of dill or chives for extra flavor.
For a crunchier texture, include cucumber slices or radish.
N.V.: Calories: 320, Fat: 23g, Carbs: 8g, Protein: 22g, Sugar: 2g

BALANCED LUNCH OPTIONS

1. ROASTED CHICKPEA AND QUINOA SALAD

P.T.: 15 min
C.T.: 30 min
M.C.: Roasting & Simmering
SERVINGS: 4
INGR.:
1 cup quinoa
2 cups vegetable broth
1 can (15 oz) chickpeas, drained, rinsed, and dried
1 Tblsp olive oil
1/2 tsp smoked paprika
1/4 tsp garlic powder
Salt and pepper to taste
2 cups arugula
1 cup cherry tomatoes, halved
1/2 cucumber, diced
1/4 cup feta cheese, crumbled

For the dressing:
3 Tblsp olive oil
1 Tblsp lemon juice
1 tsp honey
1/4 tsp salt
1/8 tsp black pepper
DIRECTIONS:
Preheat oven to 425°F (220°C).
On a baking sheet, toss chickpeas with 1 Tblsp olive oil, smoked paprika, garlic powder, salt, and pepper. Roast for 25-30 minutes until crispy.
In a saucepan, bring quinoa and vegetable broth to a boil. Reduce heat, cover, and simmer for 15 minutes. Let it sit covered for 5 minutes, then fluff with a fork.

In a large bowl, mix the cooked quinoa, roasted chickpeas, arugula, cherry tomatoes, cucumber, and feta cheese.

Whisk together dressing ingredients and pour over the salad. Toss to combine.

TIPS:

For a vegan option, substitute feta cheese with a vegan cheese or omit.

Add avocado slices for extra creaminess and healthy fats.

N.V.: Calories: 380, Fat: 18g, Carbs: 45g, Protein: 12g, Sugar: 6g

2. TURKEY AND AVOCADO WRAP

P.T.: 10 min
C.T.: 0 min
M.C.: Wrapping
SERVINGS: 2
INGR.:

2 whole wheat tortillas
6 oz sliced turkey breast
1 ripe avocado, sliced
1/2 cup baby spinach
1/4 cup shredded carrot
2 Tblsp hummus
Salt and pepper to taste

DIRECTIONS:

Spread 1 Tblsp of hummus on each tortilla.

Layer turkey slices, avocado slices, baby spinach, and shredded carrot on top of the hummus.

Season with salt and pepper.

Roll up the tortillas tightly, slice in half, and serve.

TIPS:

For a gluten-free option, use gluten-free tortillas.

Sprinkle with a pinch of chili flakes for added spice.

N.V.: Calories: 320, Fat: 15g, Carbs: 27g, Protein: 20g, Sugar: 3g

3. SPINACH AND GOAT CHEESE STUFFED CHICKEN

P.T.: 20 min
C.T.: 25 min
M.C.: Baking
SERVINGS: 4
INGR.:

4 boneless, skinless chicken breasts
1 cup fresh spinach, chopped
1/2 cup goat cheese, crumbled
2 Tblsp olive oil
Salt and pepper to taste
1 tsp dried basil
1 tsp garlic powder

DIRECTIONS:

Preheat oven to 375°F (190°C).

Cut a pocket into the side of each chicken breast. Stuff with spinach and goat cheese. Secure with toothpicks.

Rub chicken with olive oil and season with salt, pepper, basil, and garlic powder.

Place chicken in a baking dish and bake for 25 minutes, or until chicken is cooked through.

TIPS:

Serve with a side of roasted vegetables for a complete meal.

For added flavor, marinate chicken breasts in a mixture of olive oil and lemon juice before stuffing.

N.V.: Calories: 290, Fat: 14g, Carbs: 2g, Protein: 38g, Sugar: 1g

---

4. LEMON HERB TILAPIA OVER KALE AND QUINOA SALAD

P.T.: 15 min
C.T.: 12 min
M.C.: Baking & Boiling
SERVINGS: 4
INGR.:
4 tilapia fillets
2 Tblsp lemon juice
1 Tblsp olive oil
1 tsp dried oregano
1 tsp dried thyme
Salt and pepper to taste
1 cup quinoa
2 cups water
4 cups kale, chopped
1/4 cup dried cranberries
1/4 cup sliced almonds

DIRECTIONS:

Preheat oven to 400°F (204°C).

Place tilapia fillets on a baking sheet. Mix lemon juice, olive oil, oregano, thyme, salt, and pepper. Brush over fillets.

Bake for 12 minutes or until fish flakes easily with a fork.

Meanwhile, cook quinoa in water as directed on package. Fluff and let cool.

Toss cooled quinoa with kale, cranberries, and almonds.

Serve tilapia over the kale and quinoa salad.

TIPS:

Massage kale with a little olive oil and lemon juice to soften.

Add feta cheese to the salad for a creamy texture.

N.V.: Calories: 350, Fat: 10g, Carbs: 38g, Protein: 32g, Sugar: 5g

WHOLESOME DINNERS

1. HERB-CRUSTED SALMON WITH LENTILS

P.T.: 15 min
C.T.: 20 min
M.C.: Baking & Simmering
SERVINGS: 4
INGR.:

4 salmon fillets (6 oz each)
2 Tblsp Dijon mustard
1/4 cup panko breadcrumbs
1/4 cup fresh parsley, finely chopped
2 Tblsp fresh dill, finely chopped

Salt and pepper to taste

1 cup green lentils, rinsed

2 cups vegetable broth

1 bay leaf

1/2 red onion, diced

1 carrot, diced

1 Tblsp olive oil

DIRECTIONS:

Preheat oven to 400°F (204°C). Place salmon fillets on a baking sheet. Spread Dijon mustard over the tops of the fillets.

In a small bowl, mix panko, parsley, dill, salt, and pepper. Press the panko mixture onto the mustard-coated salmon.

Bake for 15-20 minutes, or until the crust is golden and salmon flakes easily with a fork.

Meanwhile, in a saucepan, combine lentils, vegetable broth, bay leaf, red onion, carrot, and a pinch of salt. Bring to a boil, then simmer covered for 20 minutes, or until lentils are tender.

Serve the herb-crusted salmon over a bed of the cooked lentils.

TIPS:

Squeeze lemon juice over the salmon before serving for added zest.

Remove the bay leaf from lentils before serving.

N.V.: Calories: 460, Fat: 18g, Carbs: 39g, Protein: 39g, Sugar: 3g

2. STUFFED ACORN SQUASH

P.T.: 20 min

C.T.: 40 min

M.C.: Baking & Sautéing

SERVINGS: 4

INGR.:

2 acorn squash, halved and seeded

1 lb ground turkey

1 Tblsp olive oil

1/2 cup quinoa

1 cup chicken broth

1 small onion, diced

2 cloves garlic, minced

1 tsp ground cumin

1 tsp smoked paprika

Salt and pepper to taste

1/2 cup dried cranberries

1/4 cup pecans, chopped

Fresh parsley, for garnish

DIRECTIONS:

Preheat oven to 375°F (190°C). Place squash halves cut-side up on a baking sheet. Drizzle with olive oil and season with salt and pepper. Bake for 30-40 minutes, or until tender.

While squash is baking, cook quinoa in chicken broth according to package instructions. Set aside.

In a skillet, heat olive oil over medium heat. Sauté onion and garlic until translucent. Add ground turkey, cumin, smoked paprika, salt, and pepper. Cook until turkey is browned.

Stir in cooked quinoa, dried cranberries, and pecans. Cook for an additional 5 minutes.

Stuff the baked acorn squash with the turkey and quinoa mixture. Return to the oven for 10 minutes.

Garnish with fresh parsley before serving.

TIPS:

Substitute ground turkey with a plant-based protein for a vegetarian option.

Drizzle with a balsamic reduction for added flavor.

N.V.: Calories: 450, Fat: 15g, Carbs: 55g, Protein: 25g, Sugar: 15g

3. LEMON GARLIC SHRIMP WITH ZUCCHINI NOODLES

P.T.: 10 min
C.T.: 10 min
M.C.: Sautéing
SERVINGS: 4
INGR.:

1 lb large shrimp, peeled and deveined
3 Tblsp olive oil
4 cloves garlic, minced
1 lemon, juice and zest
Salt and pepper to taste
4 zucchinis, spiralized
1/4 cup fresh parsley, chopped
Red pepper flakes, optional

DIRECTIONS:

Heat 2 Tblsp olive oil in a large skillet over medium-high heat. Add garlic and sauté until fragrant.

Add shrimp to the skillet, season with salt and pepper, and cook until pink and opaque. Stir in lemon juice and zest. Remove shrimp from skillet and set aside.

In the same skillet, add the remaining olive oil and zucchini noodles. Sauté for 2-3 minutes, until just tender.

Return shrimp to the skillet with the zucchini noodles. Toss to combine.

Garnish with parsley and red pepper flakes if desired.

TIPS:

Avoid overcooking the zucchini noodles to maintain a slightly crunchy texture.

Serve with grated Parmesan cheese for added flavor.

N.V.: Calories: 290, Fat: 12g, Carbs: 10g, Protein: 35g, Sugar: 5g

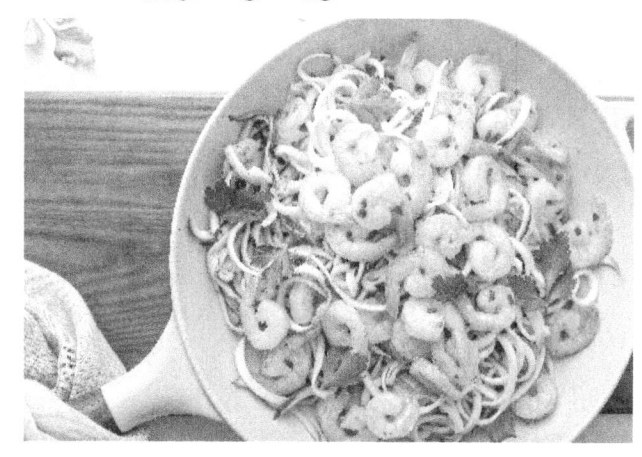

4. CREAMY MUSHROOM AND SPINACH RISOTTO

P.T.: 10 min
C.T.: 25 min
M.C.: Stirring
SERVINGS: 4

INGR.:

1 cup Arborio rice

2 Tblsp olive oil

1 small onion, diced

2 cloves garlic, minced

1/2 lb cremini mushrooms, sliced

4 cups vegetable broth, warmed

2 cups fresh spinach

1/2 cup Parmesan cheese, grated

Salt and pepper to taste

1/4 cup heavy cream

DIRECTIONS:

In a large pan, heat olive oil over medium heat. Add onion and garlic, sautéing until soft.

Add mushrooms and cook until they release their moisture and begin to brown.

Stir in Arborio rice, toasting for 1-2 minutes. Gradually add broth, 1 cup at a time, stirring constantly. Wait until each addition is absorbed before adding the next.

Once rice is tender and creamy, stir in spinach, Parmesan, and heavy cream. Season with salt and pepper. Cook until spinach is wilted.

TIPS:

For a vegan version, substitute Parmesan cheese with nutritional yeast and use coconut cream.

Garnish with additional Parmesan and fresh cracked black pepper.

N.V.: Calories: 410, Fat: 18g, Carbs: 50g, Protein: 12g

SNACKS FOR ENERGY BALANCE

1. CRUNCHY KALE CHIPS

P.T.: 10 min

C.T.: 15 min

M.C.: Baking

SERVINGS: 4

INGR.:

1 bunch kale, washed and dried

1 Tblsp olive oil

1/4 tsp salt

1/4 tsp garlic powder

DIRECTIONS:

Preheat oven to 300°F (150°C). Tear kale leaves into bite-size pieces, discarding the stems.

Toss kale pieces with olive oil, salt, and garlic powder in a large bowl until evenly coated.

Spread kale in a single layer on a baking sheet lined with parchment paper.

Bake for 15 minutes, or until crisp, turning halfway through.

TIPS:

For extra flavor, sprinkle with nutritional yeast before baking.

Store in an airtight container to keep them crispy.

N.V.: Calories: 58, Fat: 3.5g, Carbs: 6g, Protein: 2g, Sugar: 0g

2. ALMOND BUTTER ENERGY BITES

P.T.: 15 min
C.T.: 0 min
M.C.: No cook
SERVINGS: 12 bites
INGR.:

1 cup rolled oats
1/2 cup almond butter
1/4 cup honey
1/4 cup flaxseed meal
1/4 cup dark chocolate chips
1 tsp vanilla extract
Pinch of salt

DIRECTIONS:

In a large bowl, mix together oats, almond butter, honey, flaxseed meal, chocolate chips, vanilla extract, and salt until well combined.

Roll the mixture into 12 bite-sized balls.

Refrigerate for at least 30 minutes before serving to allow them to set.

TIPS:

For added protein, mix in a scoop of your favorite protein powder.

Substitute almond butter with peanut or cashew butter if preferred.

N.V.: Calories: 150, Fat: 8g, Carbs: 17g, Protein: 4g, Sugar: 9g

3. SPICY ROASTED CHICKPEAS

P.T.: 5 min
C.T.: 30 min
M.C.: Roasting
SERVINGS: 4
INGR.:

1 can (15 oz) chickpeas, drained, rinsed, and dried
1 Tblsp olive oil
1/2 tsp chili powder
1/4 tsp cumin
1/4 tsp paprika
Salt to taste

DIRECTIONS:

Preheat oven to 400°F (204°C).

Toss chickpeas with olive oil, chili powder, cumin, paprika, and salt.

Spread on a baking sheet in a single layer.

Roast for 30 minutes, shaking the pan halfway through, until crispy.

TIPS:

Serve as a salad topping for extra crunch.

Adjust spice levels to taste.

N.V.: Calories: 134, Fat: 6g, Carbs: 16g, Protein: 5g, Sugar: 0g

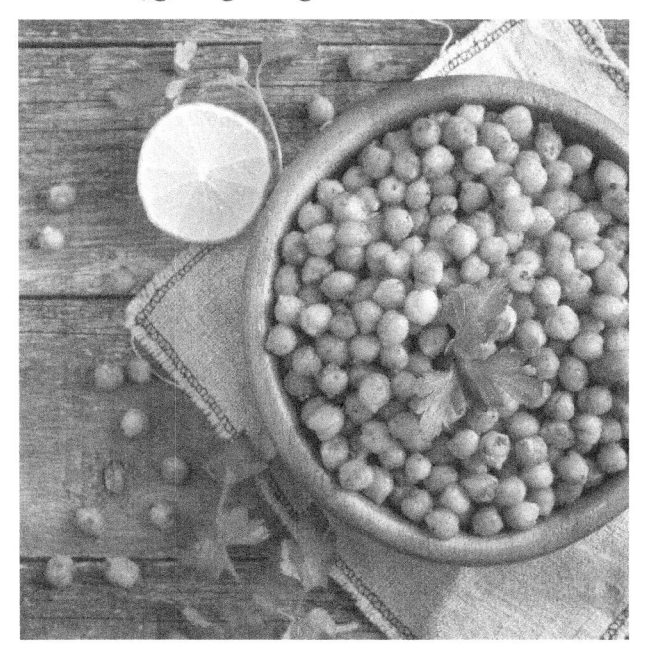

4. AVOCADO AND COTTAGE CHEESE STUFFED BELL PEPPERS

P.T.: 10 min

C.T.: 0 min

M.C.: No cook

SERVINGS: 2

INGR.:

2 bell peppers, halved and seeded

1/2 cup cottage cheese

1 avocado, diced

1/4 cup cherry tomatoes, quartered

2 Tblsp red onion, minced

1 Tblsp lime juice

Salt and pepper to taste

Cilantro for garnish

DIRECTIONS:

In a bowl, mix cottage cheese, avocado, cherry tomatoes, red onion, lime juice, salt, and pepper.

Fill each bell pepper half with the mixture.

Garnish with cilantro before serving.

TIPS:

Chill before serving for a refreshing snack.

Add a dash of hot sauce for a spicy kick.

N.V.: Calories: 220, Fat: 15g, Carbs: 18g, Protein: 9g, Sugar: 6g

5. GREEK YOGURT AND BERRY PARFAIT

P.T.: 5 min

C.T.: 0 min

M.C.: Layering

SERVINGS: 2

INGR.:

1 cup Greek yogurt

1/2 cup mixed berries (strawberries, blueberries, raspberries)

1/4 cup granola

1 Tblsp honey

Mint leaves for garnish

DIRECTIONS:

In serving glasses, layer Greek yogurt, mixed berries, and granola. Repeat layers until ingredients are used up.

Drizzle with honey and garnish with mint leaves.

TIPS:

Use honey or maple syrup for added sweetness.

Substitute with any seasonal fruits available.

N.V.: Calories: 190, Fat: 2g, Carbs: 35g, Protein: 10g, Sugar: 20g

6. CUCUMBER HUMMUS BITES

P.T.: 10 min

C.T.: 0 min

M.C.: Assembling

SERVINGS: 4

INGR.:

2 large cucumbers, sliced into thick rounds

1 cup hummus

Paprika for sprinkling

Black sesame seeds for garnish

DIRECTIONS:

Spread a dollop of hummus on each cucumber round.

Sprinkle with paprika and garnish with black sesame seeds.

TIPS:

For a variation, top with diced red peppers or olives.

Chill the cucumbers before assembling for a refreshing snack.

N.V.: Calories: 90, Fat: 5g, Carbs: 9g, Protein: 5g, Sugar: 2g

CHAPTER 6: RECIPES FOR MUSCLE GAIN
PROTEIN-PACKED BREAKFASTS

1. SPINACH AND FETA PROTEIN MUFFINS

P.T.: 15 min
C.T.: 20 min
M.C.: Baking
SERVINGS: 6
INGR.:
6 large eggs
1 cup fresh spinach, chopped
1/2 cup feta cheese, crumbled
1/4 cup red bell pepper, finely diced
1/4 cup onions, finely diced
Salt and pepper to taste
Cooking spray
DIRECTIONS:
Preheat oven to 375°F (190°C). Spray a muffin tin with cooking spray.
In a bowl, whisk together eggs, spinach, feta cheese, red bell pepper, onions, salt, and pepper.
Pour the mixture evenly into the muffin tins.
Bake for 20 minutes, or until the tops are firm to the touch and eggs are cooked.
TIPS:
Serve with a side of salsa for extra flavor.
Can be stored in the refrigerator for up to 4 days for an easy grab-and-go breakfast.
N.V.: Calories: 140, Fat: 9g, Carbs: 3g, Protein: 12g, Sugar: 2g

2. QUINOA AND EGG BREAKFAST BOWL

P.T.: 5 min
C.T.: 20 min
M.C.: Boiling & Sautéing
SERVINGS: 4
INGR.:
1 cup quinoa
2 cups water
4 large eggs
1 avocado, sliced
1 cup cherry tomatoes, halved
1/4 cup green onions, sliced
Salt and pepper to taste
1 Tblsp olive oil
DIRECTIONS:
Rinse quinoa under cold water. In a medium pot, bring quinoa and water to a boil. Reduce to a simmer, cover, and cook until all water is absorbed, about 15 minutes.
While quinoa is cooking, heat olive oil in a skillet. Crack eggs into the skillet, and cook to your preference.
Divide the cooked quinoa among four bowls. Top each with a fried egg, avocado slices, cherry tomatoes, and green onions. Season with salt and pepper.
TIPS:
Drizzle with hot sauce or salsa for added flavor.

Substitute quinoa with brown rice or farro for variety.

N.V.: Calories: 310, Fat: 15g, Carbs: 32g, Protein: 13g, Sugar: 1g

3. TURKEY SAUSAGE AND SWEET POTATO SKILLET

P.T.: 10 min
C.T.: 25 min
M.C.: Sautéing
SERVINGS: 4
INGR.:
1 lb lean turkey sausage, removed from casings
2 medium sweet potatoes, diced
1 bell pepper, diced
1 onion, diced
2 cloves garlic, minced
1 tsp smoked paprika
Salt and pepper to taste
4 large eggs
1 Tblsp olive oil
DIRECTIONS:
Heat olive oil in a large skillet over medium heat. Add turkey sausage and cook until browned. Remove and set aside.
In the same skillet, add sweet potatoes, bell pepper, and onion. Cook until vegetables are soft, about 15 minutes.
Add garlic, smoked paprika, salt, and pepper. Return sausage to the skillet and mix well.
Make four wells in the mixture and crack an egg into each. Cover and cook until eggs are set.

TIPS:
Garnish with fresh parsley or chives for added color and flavor.
For a spicier version, add red pepper flakes when cooking the vegetables.

N.V.: Calories: 350, Fat: 18g, Carbs: 25g, Protein: 24g, Sugar: 5g

4. GREEK YOGURT OAT PANCAKES

P.T.: 10 min
C.T.: 10 min
M.C.: Griddling
SERVINGS: 4
INGR.:
2 cups rolled oats
1 cup Greek yogurt
4 large eggs
1 banana, mashed
1 tsp baking powder
1/2 tsp cinnamon
1 tsp vanilla extract
Cooking spray
DIRECTIONS:
Blend oats in a food processor until they reach a flour-like consistency.
In a large bowl, mix blended oats, Greek yogurt, eggs, mashed banana, baking powder, cinnamon, and vanilla extract until smooth.
Heat a skillet over medium heat and spray

with cooking spray. Pour 1/4 cup of batter for each pancake. Cook until bubbles form, then flip and cook until golden brown.

TIPS:

Serve with a dollop of Greek yogurt and fresh berries on top.

Add a scoop of protein powder to the batter for an extra protein boost.

N.V.: Calories: 290, Fat: 8g, Carbs: 38g, Protein: 17g, Sugar: 7g

5. CHICKEN AND EGG BREAKFAST BURRITO

P.T.: 15 min
C.T.: 10 min
M.C.: Sautéing & Wrapping
SERVINGS: 4
INGR.:

4 whole wheat tortillas

1 lb cooked chicken breast, shredded

4 large eggs, beaten

1/2 cup black beans, rinsed and drained

1/2 cup shredded cheddar cheese

1 avocado, sliced

1/4 cup salsa

Salt and pepper to taste

1 Tblsp olive oil

DIRECTIONS:

Heat olive oil in a skillet over medium heat. Add eggs and cook, scrambling until set.

Lay out tortillas on a flat surface. Divide the scrambled eggs, chicken, black beans, cheddar cheese, and avocado slices evenly among the tortillas.

Roll up each tortilla, folding in the sides to enclose the filling. Serve with salsa on the side.

TIPS:

For a vegetarian option, substitute chicken with extra firm tofu.

Warm the tortillas before assembling for easier rolling.

N.V.: Calories: 420, Fat: 20g, Carbs: 32g, Protein: 34g, Sugar: 3g

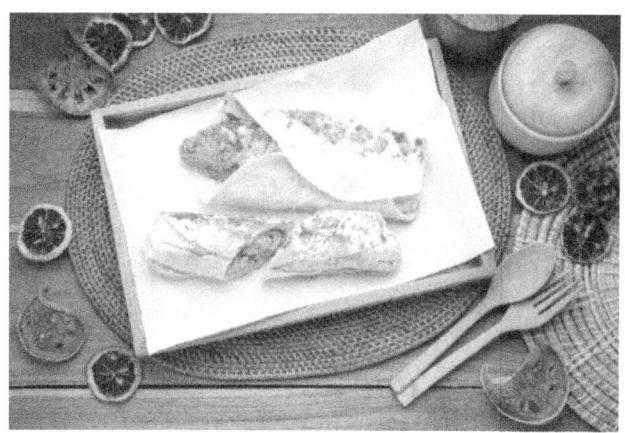

POST-WORKOUT LUNCHES

1. GRILLED CHICKEN AND QUINOA SALAD

P.T.: 15 min
C.T.: 15 min
M.C.: Grilling & Boiling
SERVINGS: 4
INGR.:

4 chicken breasts (6 oz each)

1 cup quinoa

2 cups water

2 avocados, diced

1 cup cherry tomatoes, halved

1/4 cup red onion, finely chopped

2 Tblsp olive oil

Juice of 1 lemon

Salt and pepper to taste

1/4 cup fresh cilantro, chopped

DIRECTIONS:

Season chicken breasts with salt and pepper, brush with 1 Tblsp olive oil, and grill over medium-high heat for 7-8 minutes per side or until fully cooked. Let rest for 5 minutes, then slice.

Rinse quinoa under cold water. In a medium pot, bring quinoa and water to a boil, reduce heat to low, cover, and simmer for 15 minutes or until water is absorbed. Fluff with a fork and let cool.

In a large bowl, combine cooled quinoa, sliced chicken, avocados, cherry tomatoes, red onion, lemon juice, remaining olive oil, salt, pepper, and cilantro. Toss until evenly mixed.

TIPS:

For a zesty flavor, add the zest of the lemon to the salad.

Serve over a bed of mixed greens for added nutrients.

N.V.: Calories: 490, Fat: 22g, Carbs: 40g, Protein: 35g, Sugar: 4g

2. TUNA AND CHICKPEA PITA POCKETS

P.T.: 10 min

C.T.: 0 min

M.C.: Assembly

SERVINGS: 4

INGR.:

2 cans (5 oz each) tuna in water, drained

1 can (15 oz) chickpeas, rinsed and drained

1/4 cup Greek yogurt

1/2 cucumber, diced

1/4 cup red onion, finely chopped

2 Tblsp fresh dill, chopped

Juice of 1 lemon

Salt and pepper to taste

4 whole wheat pita breads, halved

DIRECTIONS:

In a bowl, mix tuna, chickpeas, Greek yogurt, cucumber, red onion, dill, lemon juice, salt, and pepper until well combined.

Gently open pita halves and fill with the tuna mixture.

TIPS:

Add a handful of spinach or arugula to each pita pocket for extra greens.

For a dairy-free option, substitute Greek yogurt with avocado.

N.V.: Calories: 320, Fat: 6g, Carbs: 45g, Protein: 25g, Sugar: 6g

3. SWEET POTATO AND BLACK BEAN BURRITO BOWL

P.T.: 20 min
C.T.: 25 min
M.C.: Roasting & Boiling
SERVINGS: 4
INGR.:

2 large sweet potatoes, cubed
1 Tblsp olive oil
1 tsp cumin
1 tsp paprika
Salt and pepper to taste
1 cup brown rice
2 cups water
1 can (15 oz) black beans, drained and rinsed
1 avocado, sliced
1/4 cup fresh cilantro, chopped
Juice of 1 lime

DIRECTIONS:

Preheat oven to 425°F (220°C). Toss sweet potatoes with olive oil, cumin, paprika, salt, and pepper. Spread on a baking sheet and roast for 25 minutes, until tender.

Rinse brown rice under cold water. In a pot, bring brown rice and water to a boil, reduce heat, cover, and simmer for 45 minutes or until water is absorbed.

In bowls, layer cooked rice, roasted sweet potatoes, black beans, and avocado slices. Garnish with cilantro and drizzle with lime juice.

TIPS:

Add grilled chicken or tofu for extra protein.
Drizzle with a homemade or store-bought salsa verde for added flavor.

N.V.: Calories: 430, Fat: 10g, Carbs: 74g, Protein: 14g, Sugar: 7g

4. EGGS AND TURKEY BACON ON WHOLE GRAIN TOAST

P.T.: 5 min
C.T.: 10 min
M.C.: Pan-frying & Toasting
SERVINGS: 4
INGR.:

8 slices of turkey bacon
8 large eggs
4 slices of whole grain bread
Salt and pepper to taste
Cooking spray

DIRECTIONS:

Cook turkey bacon in a skillet over medium heat until crisp. Set aside on paper towels.

In the same skillet, spray cooking spray, and fry eggs to your liking. Season with salt and pepper.

Toast whole grain bread and place two slices of turkey bacon and two eggs on each slice.

TIPS:

Top with avocado slices or a sprinkle of cheese for extra flavor.
Add a side of sautéed spinach or tomatoes for added vegetables.

N.V.: Calories: 330, Fat: 14g, Carbs: 23g, Protein: 27g, Sugar: 3g

5. PROTEIN-PACKED SMOOTHIE

P.T.: 5 min

C.T.: 0 min

M.C.: Blending

SERVINGS: 2

INGR.:

1 cup unsweetened almond milk

1 banana, frozen

1/2 cup Greek yogurt

2 Tblsp peanut butter

1 scoop protein powder

1 Tblsp chia seeds

1 Tblsp honey

Ice cubes

DIRECTIONS:

Combine all ingredients in a blender. Blend on high until smooth and creamy.

Adjust sweetness with more honey if desired and blend again. Serve immediately.

TIPS:

Use a vanilla or chocolate protein powder for added flavor.

Top with a sprinkle of granola for crunch.

N.V.: Calories: 350, Fat: 14g, Carbs: 34g, Protein: 25g, Sugar: 18g

MUSCLE-BUILDING DINNERS

1. BEEF AND BROCCOLI STIR-FRY

P.T.: 10 min

C.T.: 15 min

M.C.: Stir-frying

SERVINGS: 4

INGR.:

1 lb lean beef steak, thinly sliced

2 cups broccoli florets

1 red bell pepper, sliced

2 Tblsp olive oil

2 cloves garlic, minced

For the sauce:

1/4 cup soy sauce

2 Tblsp oyster sauce

1 Tblsp honey

1 tsp ginger, grated

1 Tblsp cornstarch

1/2 cup water

DIRECTIONS:

In a small bowl, whisk together the soy sauce, oyster sauce, honey, ginger, cornstarch, and water. Set aside.

Heat olive oil in a large skillet or wok over medium-high heat. Add garlic and stir-fry for 30 seconds.

Add beef slices and stir-fry for 2-3 minutes, or until they start to brown.

Add broccoli and bell pepper, continue to stir-fry for another 5 minutes.

Pour the sauce over the beef and vegetables, stirring continuously until the sauce thickens and everything is well coated.

TIPS:

Serve over brown rice or quinoa for added fiber and nutrients.

Sprinkle with sesame seeds before serving for a nutty flavor.

N.V.: Calories: 280, Fat: 14g, Carbs: 15g, Protein: 26g, Sugar: 5g

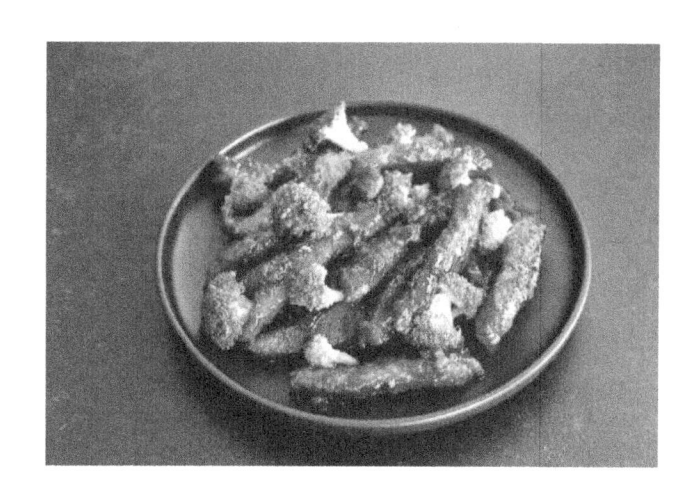

2. SALMON WITH QUINOA AND SPINACH SALAD

P.T.: 15 min
C.T.: 20 min
M.C.: Baking & Boiling
SERVINGS: 4
INGR.:
4 salmon fillets (6 oz each)
1 cup quinoa
2 cups water
4 cups fresh spinach
1/4 cup dried cranberries
1/4 cup slivered almonds
2 Tblsp olive oil
Salt and pepper to taste
Lemon wedges for serving

DIRECTIONS:
Preheat oven to 375°F (190°C). Season salmon with salt and pepper, place on a baking sheet, and drizzle with 1 Tblsp olive oil. Bake for 15-20 minutes, or until salmon flakes easily with a fork.

Rinse quinoa under cold water. In a pot, bring quinoa and water to a boil, reduce heat, cover, and simmer for 15 minutes or until water is absorbed.

In a large bowl, toss cooked quinoa, spinach, dried cranberries, almonds, and remaining olive oil. Season with salt and pepper to taste. Serve salmon over the quinoa and spinach salad, with lemon wedges on the side.

TIPS:
Add avocado slices to the salad for healthy fats.

For a citrusy flavor, zest the lemon over the salmon before baking.

N.V.: Calories: 500, Fat: 22g, Carbs: 45g, Protein: 35g, Sugar: 8g

3. TURKEY MEATBALLS WITH SPAGHETTI SQUASH

P.T.: 20 min
C.T.: 40 min
M.C.: Baking & Roasting
SERVINGS: 4

INGR.:
1 large spaghetti squash
1 lb ground turkey
1/4 cup breadcrumbs

1/4 cup Parmesan cheese, grated

1 egg

2 cloves garlic, minced

1 tsp Italian seasoning

Salt and pepper to taste

2 cups marinara sauce

DIRECTIONS:

Preheat oven to 400°F (204°C). Halve the spaghetti squash lengthwise and scoop out the seeds. Place cut-side down on a baking sheet and roast for 40 minutes.

In a bowl, mix ground turkey, breadcrumbs, Parmesan, egg, garlic, Italian seasoning, salt, and pepper. Form into 1-inch meatballs.

Place meatballs on a greased baking sheet and bake for 20 minutes, or until cooked through.

Use a fork to shred the cooked squash into "spaghetti." Serve meatballs and marinara sauce over the spaghetti squash.

TIPS:

For a lower calorie option, use ground turkey breast.

Garnish with fresh basil for added flavor.

N.V.: Calories: 330, Fat: 14g, Carbs: 28g, Protein: 27g, Sugar: 8g

4. GRILLED STEAK WITH SWEET POTATO FRIES

P.T.: 10 min
C.T.: 30 min
M.C.: Grilling & Baking
SERVINGS: 4
INGR.:

4 beef steaks (6 oz each)

2 large sweet potatoes, cut into fries

2 Tblsp olive oil

Salt and pepper to taste

1 tsp paprika

1 tsp garlic powder

DIRECTIONS:

Preheat grill to high heat and oven to 425°F (220°C).

Toss sweet potato fries with 1 Tblsp olive oil, salt, pepper, paprika, and garlic powder. Spread on a baking sheet and bake for 25-30 minutes, turning halfway, until crispy.

Season steaks with salt and pepper. Grill for 4-5 minutes per side for medium-rare, or to desired doneness. Let rest for 5 minutes before slicing.

Serve grilled steaks with sweet potato fries on the side.

TIPS:

For extra flavor, marinate steaks in your favorite steak seasoning for at least 30 minutes before grilling.

Serve with a side of steamed vegetables for a balanced meal.

N.V.: Calories: 520, Fat: 22g, Carbs: 38g, Protein: 46g, Sugar: 6g

RECOVERY SNACKS

1. COTTAGE CHEESE AND PEAR PARFAIT

P.T.: 5 min
C.T.: 0 min
M.C.: Layering
SERVINGS: 2
INGR.:
1 cup low-fat cottage cheese
1 pear, diced
1/4 cup granola
1 Tblsp honey
1/2 tsp cinnamon
DIRECTIONS:

In two serving glasses, layer half of the cottage cheese, diced pear, and granola. Repeat the layers.

Drizzle honey over the top and sprinkle with cinnamon before serving.

TIPS:

For added texture, include a handful of chopped walnuts or almonds.

Substitute pear with any seasonal fruit of your choice for variety.

N.V.: Calories: 220, Fat: 2g, Carbs: 35g, Protein: 15g, Sugar: 20g

2. AVOCADO CHOCOLATE MOUSSE

P.T.: 10 min
C.T.: 0 min
M.C.: Blending
SERVINGS: 4
INGR.:
2 ripe avocados, peeled and pitted
1/4 cup cocoa powder
1/4 cup maple syrup
1/2 tsp vanilla extract
Pinch of salt
Berries for garnish
DIRECTIONS:

In a blender, combine avocados, cocoa powder, maple syrup, vanilla extract, and a pinch of salt. Blend until smooth.

Divide the mousse into serving dishes and refrigerate for at least 1 hour.

Garnish with berries before serving.

TIPS:

For a richer flavor, add a tablespoon of peanut butter to the blend.

Ensure the mousse is chilled well to enhance its texture and flavor.

N.V.: Calories: 240, Fat: 15g, Carbs: 27g, Protein: 4g, Sugar: 15g

3. GREEK YOGURT WITH HOMEMADE GRANOLA

P.T.: 15 min
C.T.: 30 min
M.C.: Baking

SERVINGS: 4
INGREDIENTS for Granola:
2 cups rolled oats

1/2 cup chopped almonds

1/4 cup pumpkin seeds

1/4 cup honey

2 Tblsp coconut oil, melted

1/2 tsp vanilla extract

1/2 tsp cinnamon

Pinch of salt

For Serving:

2 cups Greek yogurt

Fresh berries

DIRECTIONS:

Preheat oven to 300°F (150°C). Mix oats, almonds, pumpkin seeds, honey, coconut oil, vanilla, cinnamon, and salt. Spread on a baking sheet.

Bake for 30 minutes, stirring occasionally, until golden brown. Let cool.

Serve granola over Greek yogurt, topped with fresh berries.

TIPS:

Store leftover granola in an airtight container for up to 2 weeks.

Add dried fruit to the granola after baking for added sweetness.

N.V.: Calories: 350, Fat: 14g, Carbs: 44g, Protein: 17g, Sugar: 18g

4. PROTEIN PEANUT BUTTER BANANA SMOOTHIE

P.T.: 5 min

C.T.: 0 min

M.C.: Blending

SERVINGS: 2

INGR.:

2 bananas, frozen

2 Tblsp peanut butter

1 cup almond milk

1 scoop protein powder

Ice cubes

DIRECTIONS:

Combine bananas, peanut butter, almond milk, protein powder, and ice cubes in a blender.

Blend until smooth and creamy. Serve immediately.

TIPS:

For added nutrition, include a tablespoon of flaxseed or chia seeds.

Adjust the thickness by adding more or less almond milk.

N.V.: Calories: 320, Fat: 10g, Carbs: 38g, Protein: 25g, Sugar: 20g

5. SWEET POTATO PROTEIN BROWNIES

P.T.: 20 min

C.T.: 25 min

M.C.: Baking

SERVINGS: 8

INGR.:

1 large sweet potato, cooked and mashed

1/2 cup almond butter

2 Tblsp cocoa powder

1/4 cup maple syrup

1 scoop chocolate protein powder

1 tsp vanilla extract

1/2 tsp baking powder

Pinch of salt

DIRECTIONS:

Preheat oven to 350°F (175°C). Mix all ingredients in a bowl until well combined. Pour the mixture into a greased 8x8 inch baking dish.

Bake for 25 minutes, or until a toothpick comes out clean. Let cool before slicing.

TIPS:

Serve with a dollop of Greek yogurt for extra protein.

Store in an airtight container in the fridge for up to 5 days.

N.V.: Calories: 200, Fat: 10g, Carbs: 20g, Protein: 10g, Sugar: 10g

6. ALMOND JOY PROTEIN BALLS

P.T.: 15 min

C.T.: 0 min

M.C.: No cook

SERVINGS: 12 balls

INGR.:

1 cup rolled oats

1/2 cup almond butter

1/4 cup shredded coconut

1/4 cup chocolate chips

2 Tblsp honey

1 scoop vanilla protein powder

1 Tblsp water

DIRECTIONS:

In a bowl, mix all ingredients until well combined. If the mixture is too dry, add a little more water.

Roll the mixture into 12 balls. Place in the fridge for at least 30 minutes to set.

TIPS:

Substitute honey with maple syrup for a vegan version.

Roll balls in extra shredded coconut or cocoa powder for a decorative touch.

N.V.: Calories: 150, Fat: 8g, Carbs: 15g, Protein: 5g, Sugar: 7g

CHAPTER 7: FAT LOSS-FOCUSED RECIPES
METABOLISM-BOOSTING BREAKFASTS

1. SPICY AVOCADO TOAST WITH EGG

P.T.: 5 min
C.T.: 5 min
M.C.: Toasting & Frying
SERVINGS: 2
INGR.:
2 slices whole grain bread
1 ripe avocado
2 large eggs
1/4 tsp red pepper flakes
Salt and pepper to taste
1/2 tsp olive oil
DIRECTIONS:
Toast the bread slices to your desired crispness.
In a bowl, mash the avocado with a fork and spread it evenly on the toasted bread. Sprinkle with red pepper flakes, salt, and pepper.
Heat olive oil in a pan over medium heat. Crack the eggs into the pan and cook to your liking. Season with salt and pepper.
Place a cooked egg on top of each avocado toast. Serve immediately.
TIPS:
For added metabolism-boosting power, top with a sprinkle of turmeric.
Serve with a side of mixed greens for extra fiber.
N.V.: Calories: 290, Fat: 20g, Carbs: 20g, Protein: 12g, Sugar: 3g

2. GREEN TEA SMOOTHIE BOWL

P.T.: 10 min
C.T.: 0 min
M.C.: Blending
SERVINGS: 1
INGR.:
1 frozen banana
1/2 cup frozen spinach
1/2 cup brewed green tea, cooled
1/4 cup Greek yogurt
1 Tblsp honey
Toppings: Sliced almonds, chia seeds, fresh berries
DIRECTIONS:
In a blender, combine the frozen banana, frozen spinach, cooled green tea, Greek yogurt, and honey. Blend until smooth.
Pour the smoothie into a bowl and garnish with sliced almonds, chia seeds, and fresh berries.
TIPS:
Adjust the thickness by adding more or less green tea.
For extra protein, add a scoop of your favorite protein powder.

N.V.: Calories: 210, Fat: 2g, Carbs: 44g, Protein: 10g, Sugar: 27g

3. CINNAMON AND OATMEAL PROTEIN PANCAKES

P.T.: 10 min
C.T.: 10 min
M.C.: Griddling
SERVINGS: 4
INGR.:

1 cup rolled oats
1/2 cup cottage cheese
4 egg whites
1 tsp cinnamon
1 tsp vanilla extract
1/2 cup water
1 Tblsp maple syrup
Cooking spray

DIRECTIONS:

Blend the oats, cottage cheese, egg whites, cinnamon, vanilla extract, and water in a blender until smooth.

Heat a non-stick pan over medium heat and lightly coat with cooking spray. Pour 1/4 cup of batter for each pancake. Cook until bubbles form on the surface, then flip and cook until browned on the other side.

Serve with a drizzle of maple syrup.

TIPS:

Add blueberries or sliced bananas to the batter for extra flavor and nutrients.

Top with Greek yogurt for an additional protein boost.

N.V.: Calories: 150, Fat: 2g, Carbs: 22g, Protein: 12g, Sugar: 5g

4. TURMERIC SCRAMBLED EGGS

P.T.: 5 min
C.T.: 5 min
M.C.: Scrambling
SERVINGS: 2
INGR.:

4 large eggs
1/2 tsp turmeric
1/4 tsp black pepper
1 Tblsp milk (any kind)
Salt to taste
1/2 Tblsp olive oil
2 Tblsp chopped fresh spinach

DIRECTIONS:

In a bowl, whisk together the eggs, turmeric, black pepper, milk, and salt.

Heat olive oil in a non-stick skillet over medium heat. Add the egg mixture and chopped spinach. Cook, stirring frequently, until the eggs are scrambled and cooked through.

Serve immediately, garnished with more black pepper if desired.

TIPS:

Serve on whole grain toast for added fiber.

For an extra metabolism boost, add a pinch of cayenne pepper.

N.V.: Calories: 160, Fat: 11g, Carbs: 2g, Protein: 13g, Sugar: 1g

5. GRAPEFRUIT AND AVOCADO SALAD

P.T.: 10 min
C.T.: 0 min
M.C.: Assembling
SERVINGS: 2
INGR.:
1 large grapefruit, peeled and sectioned
1 avocado, sliced
2 cups mixed salad greens
1 Tblsp olive oil
1 Tblsp lemon juice
Salt and pepper to taste
DIRECTIONS:
On two plates, arrange the mixed salad greens. Top with grapefruit sections and avocado slices.

In a small bowl, whisk together olive oil and lemon juice. Drizzle over the salads. Season with salt and pepper to taste.

TIPS:
Add a sprinkle of chia seeds for added texture and omega-3 fatty acids.

For additional protein, top with grilled chicken or shrimp.

N.V.: Calories: 220, Fat: 15g, Carbs: 20g, Protein: 3g, Sugar: 12g

FAT-BURNING LUNCHES

1. SPINACH AND CHICKEN SALAD WITH AVOCADO DRESSING

P.T.: 15 min
C.T.: 0 min
M.C.: Assembly
SERVINGS: 4
INGR.:
2 cups cooked chicken breast, shredded
4 cups fresh spinach leaves
1 cup cherry tomatoes, halved
1/2 cucumber, sliced
1/4 red onion, thinly sliced
For the Avocado Dressing:
1 ripe avocado
1/4 cup Greek yogurt
2 Tblsp lime juice
Salt and pepper to taste
Water, as needed for consistency
DIRECTIONS:
In a large salad bowl, combine the spinach, cherry tomatoes, cucumber, red onion, and shredded chicken.

For the dressing, blend the avocado, Greek yogurt, lime juice, salt, and pepper until smooth. Add water as needed to achieve desired consistency.

Drizzle the avocado dressing over the salad and toss until everything is evenly coated.

TIPS:
For added crunch, sprinkle with toasted

almond slices or sunflower seeds. Chill the salad for 30 minutes before serving for a refreshing touch.

N.V.: Calories: 250, Fat: 8g, Carbs: 12g, Protein: 30g, Sugar: 4g

2. TURMERIC LENTIL SOUP

P.T.: 10 min
C.T.: 25 min
M.C.: Simmering
SERVINGS: 4
INGR.:
1 cup red lentils, rinsed
4 cups vegetable broth
1 carrot, diced
1 onion, diced
2 cloves garlic, minced
1 tsp turmeric
1 tsp cumin
Salt and pepper to taste
2 Tblsp olive oil
Fresh cilantro for garnish
DIRECTIONS:
Heat olive oil in a large pot over medium heat. Add onion, carrot, and garlic. Sauté until soft. Stir in turmeric, cumin, salt, and pepper, cooking for another minute until fragrant.
Add lentils and vegetable broth. Bring to a boil, then simmer for about 20 minutes or until lentils are soft.
Serve hot, garnished with fresh cilantro.
TIPS:
Squeeze a wedge of lemon into each bowl before serving for added brightness.
Serve with a side of whole grain bread for dipping.
N.V.: Calories: 230, Fat: 7g, Carbs: 30g, Protein: 12g, Sugar: 4g

3. GRILLED SALMON WITH MANGO SALSA

P.T.: 15 min
C.T.: 10 min
M.C.: Grilling
SERVINGS: 4
INGR.:
4 salmon fillets (6 oz each)
Salt and pepper to taste
1 Tblsp olive oil
For the Mango Salsa:
1 ripe mango, diced
1/2 red bell pepper, diced
1/4 red onion, finely chopped
2 Tblsp cilantro, chopped
Juice of 1 lime
Salt to taste
DIRECTIONS:
Preheat grill to medium-high heat. Season salmon with salt, pepper, and olive oil. Grill for 5 minutes on each side or until cooked through.
For the salsa, combine mango, red bell pepper, red onion, cilantro, lime juice, and

salt in a bowl. Mix well.

Serve the grilled salmon topped with mango salsa.

TIPS:

For a smoky flavor, add a pinch of smoked paprika to the salmon before grilling.

Serve with a side of mixed greens or quinoa for a complete meal.

N.V.: Calories: 320, Fat: 14g, Carbs: 16g, Protein: 34g, Sugar: 12g

4. SPICY CHICKPEA AND QUINOA BOWL

P.T.: 15 min
C.T.: 20 min
M.C.: Boiling & Roasting
SERVINGS: 4
INGR.:

1 cup quinoa

2 cups water

1 can (15 oz) chickpeas, drained and rinsed

1 tsp chili powder

1/2 tsp cumin

Salt and pepper to taste

1 avocado, sliced

1 cup cherry tomatoes, halved

1/2 cucumber, diced

1 Tblsp olive oil

Fresh lime wedges for serving

DIRECTIONS:

Preheat oven to 400°F (200°C). Toss chickpeas with chili powder, cumin, salt, pepper, and olive oil. Roast for 20 minutes, stirring halfway through.

Rinse quinoa under cold water. In a pot, bring quinoa and water to a boil, reduce heat, cover, and simmer for 15 minutes or until water is absorbed.

Assemble the bowls with cooked quinoa, roasted chickpeas, avocado slices, cherry tomatoes, and cucumber. Serve with lime wedges.

TIPS:

Add a dollop of Greek yogurt on top for creaminess and extra protein.

For more heat, drizzle with hot sauce before serving.

N.V.: Calories: 330, Fat: 12g, Carbs: 45g, Protein: 12g, Sugar: 6g

5. ZUCCHINI NOODLES WITH PESTO AND CHERRY TOMATOES

P.T.: 10 min
C.T.: 0 min
M.C.: Spiralizing
SERVINGS: 4
INGR.:

4 medium zucchinis

1 cup cherry tomatoes, halved

1/2 cup pesto

Salt and pepper to taste

Parmesan cheese, for garnish

DIRECTIONS:

Use a spiralizer to turn the zucchinis into noodles. Place in a large bowl.

Add the cherry tomatoes and pesto to the zucchini noodles. Toss until well combined.

Season with salt and pepper to taste.

Serve garnished with Parmesan cheese.

TIPS:

For added protein, top with grilled chicken or shrimp.

Squeeze a little lemon juice over the top for added zest.

N.V.: Calories: 190, Fat: 14g, Carbs: 10

LIGHT AND LEAN DINNERS

1. GRILLED TILAPIA WITH LEMON HERB QUINOA

P.T.: 10 min
C.T.: 15 min
M.C.: Grilling & Boiling
SERVINGS: 4
INGR.:

4 tilapia fillets

1 Tblsp olive oil

Salt and pepper to taste

1 lemon, sliced

1 cup quinoa

2 cups water

1 Tblsp lemon juice

1 tsp dried oregano

1 tsp dried basil

1/4 cup chopped fresh parsley

DIRECTIONS:

Preheat grill to medium-high. Brush tilapia fillets with olive oil and season with salt and pepper. Grill each side for 3-4 minutes, laying lemon slices on top while cooking.

Rinse quinoa under cold water. In a pot, combine quinoa and water, bringing to a boil. Reduce heat, cover, and simmer for 15 minutes. Fluff with a fork, then stir in lemon juice, oregano, basil, and parsley.

Serve grilled tilapia over lemon herb quinoa.

TIPS:

For added flavor, marinate the tilapia in lemon juice and herbs for 30 minutes before grilling.

Garnish with extra lemon slices and parsley before serving.

N.V.: Calories: 290, Fat: 6g, Carbs: 35g, Protein: 28g, Sugar: 1g

2. VEGGIE STUFFED BELL PEPPERS

P.T.: 15 min
C.T.: 30 min
M.C.: Baking
SERVINGS: 4

INGR.:

4 large bell peppers, tops cut off and seeds removed

1 cup cooked quinoa

1 can (15 oz) black beans, drained and rinsed

1 cup corn kernels, fresh or frozen

1/2 cup diced tomatoes

1 tsp cumin

1 tsp chili powder

Salt and pepper to taste

1/4 cup shredded low-fat cheese

DIRECTIONS:

Preheat oven to 375°F (190°C). Place bell peppers cut-side up in a baking dish.

In a bowl, mix quinoa, black beans, corn, tomatoes, cumin, chili powder, salt, and pepper. Spoon mixture into bell peppers.

Top each pepper with shredded cheese. Bake for 30 minutes, or until peppers are tender.

TIPS:

Add chopped cilantro or green onions to the filling for extra flavor.

Serve with a side of salsa or Greek yogurt for added zest and creaminess.

N.V.: Calories: 220, Fat: 3g, Carbs: 40g, Protein: 12g, Sugar: 7g

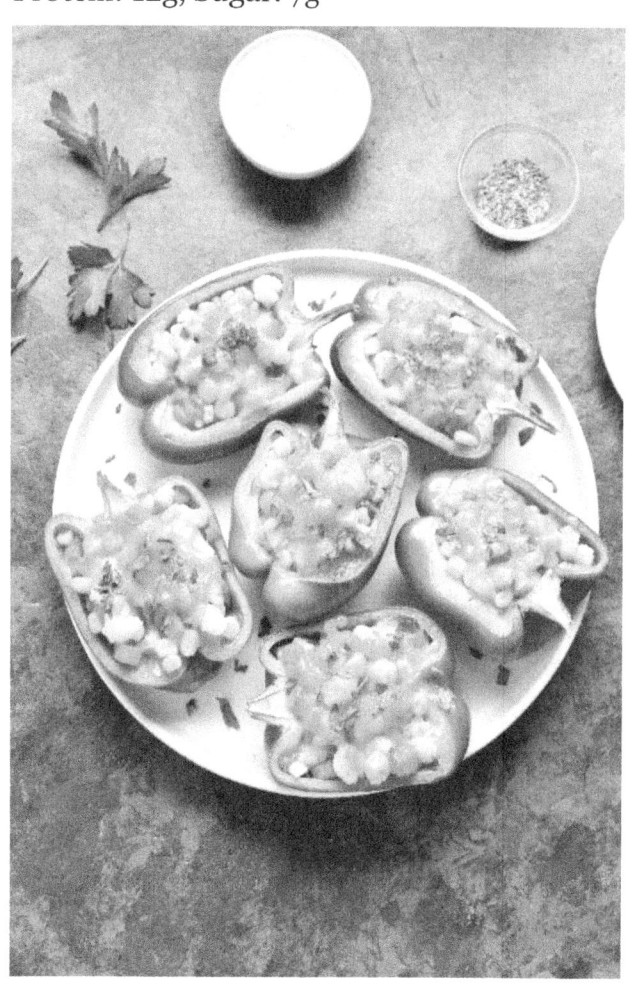

3. BAKED COD WITH SPINACH AND TOMATOES

P.T.: 10 min

C.T.: 20 min

M.C.: Baking

SERVINGS: 4

INGR.:

4 cod fillets

2 Tblsp olive oil

2 cups fresh spinach

1 cup cherry tomatoes, halved

2 cloves garlic, minced

Salt and pepper to taste

Lemon wedges for serving

DIRECTIONS:

Preheat oven to 400°F (200°C). Place cod fillets in a baking dish. Season with salt and pepper.

In a skillet, heat 1 Tblsp olive oil over medium heat. Add garlic, spinach, and tomatoes, sautéing until spinach is wilted.

Top cod with the spinach and tomato mixture. Drizzle with remaining olive oil. Bake for 20 minutes, or until cod flakes easily.

Serve with lemon wedges.

TIPS:

For added flavor, sprinkle a mix of dried herbs over the cod before baking.

Pair with a side of roasted vegetables or a quinoa salad for a complete meal.

N.V.: Calories: 200, Fat: 8g, Carbs: 6g, Protein: 28g, Sugar: 2g

4. SPICY SHRIMP AND ZUCCHINI NOODLES

P.T.: 15 min
C.T.: 10 min
M.C.: Sautéing
SERVINGS: 4
INGR.:

1 lb shrimp, peeled and deveined
4 medium zucchinis, spiralized
1 Tblsp olive oil
2 cloves garlic, minced
1 tsp red pepper flakes
Salt and pepper to taste
1/4 cup chopped fresh parsley
Lemon wedges for serving

DIRECTIONS:

Heat olive oil in a large skillet over medium heat. Add garlic and red pepper flakes, sautéing until fragrant.

Add shrimp, season with salt and pepper, and cook until pink and opaque. Remove shrimp and set aside.

In the same skillet, add spiralized zucchini. Cook for 2-3 minutes, or until tender.

Return shrimp to the skillet, tossing with zucchini noodles. Garnish with parsley. Serve with lemon wedges.

TIPS:

Avoid overcooking the zucchini noodles to maintain their texture.

For a lower calorie option, omit the olive oil and use a non-stick cooking spray.

N.V.: Calories: 180, Fat: 6g, Carbs: 8g, Protein: 24g, Sugar: 4g

LOW-CALORIE SNACKS

1. CUCUMBER ROLL-UPS WITH HUMMUS

P.T.: 10 min
C.T.: 0 min
M.C.: No cook
SERVINGS: 2
INGR.:

1 large cucumber
1/2 cup hummus
1/4 red bell pepper, finely diced
1/4 cup spinach leaves, chopped
Salt and pepper to taste

DIRECTIONS:

Slice the cucumber lengthwise into thin strips using a mandoline slicer or a vegetable peeler.

Spread a thin layer of hummus over each cucumber strip.

Sprinkle the diced bell pepper and chopped

spinach evenly over the hummus.

Carefully roll up the cucumber strips and secure them with a toothpick. Season with salt and pepper.

TIPS:

Chill the cucumber rolls before serving for a refreshing snack.

Experiment with different hummus flavors to add variety.

N.V.: Calories: 90, Fat: 5g, Carbs: 10g, Protein: 3g, Sugar: 2g

2. GREEK YOGURT AND BERRY CUPS

P.T.: 5 min
C.T.: 0 min
M.C.: No cook
SERVINGS: 4
INGR.:
2 cups Greek yogurt, low-fat
1 cup mixed berries (strawberries, blueberries, raspberries)
2 Tblsp honey
1/4 cup granola
DIRECTIONS:

In serving cups, layer Greek yogurt and mixed berries.

Drizzle honey over each cup and sprinkle with granola before serving.

TIPS:

Freeze for an hour before serving for a frozen yogurt texture.

Substitute honey with maple syrup for a vegan option.

N.V.: Calories: 150, Fat: 1g, Carbs: 22g, Protein: 12g, Sugar: 18g

3. CHILLED AVOCADO SOUP SHOTS

P.T.: 10 min
C.T.: 0 min
M.C.: Blending
SERVINGS: 4
INGR.:
2 ripe avocados
1 cup vegetable broth, chilled
1/2 cup Greek yogurt, low-fat
Juice of 1 lime
Salt and pepper to taste
1/4 cup cilantro, chopped
DIRECTIONS:

Blend avocados, vegetable broth, Greek yogurt, and lime juice until smooth.

Season with salt and pepper to taste.

Pour into shot glasses and chill until serving.

Garnish with chopped cilantro.

TIPS:

Add a dash of hot sauce for a spicy kick.

Serve as a refreshing starter for summer dinners.

N.V.: Calories: 120, Fat: 9g, Carbs: 8g, Protein: 3g, Sugar: 2g

4. CARROT AND ZUCCHINI MINI MUFFINS

P.T.: 15 min

C.T.: 20 min

M.C.: Baking

SERVINGS: 12

INGR.:

1 cup grated carrot

1 cup grated zucchini, water squeezed out

2 eggs

1/4 cup olive oil

1/4 cup honey

1 tsp vanilla extract

1 cup whole wheat flour

1 tsp baking powder

1/2 tsp cinnamon

Pinch of salt

DIRECTIONS:

Preheat oven to 350°F (175°C). Line a mini muffin tin with paper liners.

In a bowl, mix together carrot, zucchini, eggs, olive oil, honey, and vanilla.

In another bowl, whisk together flour, baking powder, cinnamon, and salt. Add to the wet ingredients, stirring until just combined.

Fill muffin tins and bake for 20 minutes or until a toothpick inserted comes out clean.

TIPS:

Let muffins cool completely on a wire rack to maintain texture.

Store in an airtight container for up to 3 days or freeze for longer storage.

N.V.: Calories: 110, Fat: 5g, Carbs: 15g, Protein: 2g, Sugar: 8g

5. SPICY ROASTED CHICKPEAS

P.T.: 5 min

C.T.: 40 min

M.C.: Roasting

SERVINGS: 4

INGR.:

1 can (15 oz) chickpeas, drained, rinsed, and dried

1 Tblsp olive oil

1/2 tsp chili powder

1/2 tsp cumin

Salt to taste

DIRECTIONS:

Preheat oven to 400°F (200°C). Toss chickpeas with olive oil, chili powder, cumin, and salt.

Spread on a baking sheet in a single layer.

Roast for 40 minutes, shaking the pan occasionally, until crispy.

TIPS:

Let chickpeas cool completely to achieve maximum crispiness.

Experiment with other spices like paprika or garlic powder for variety.

N.V.: Calories: 120, Fat: 5g, Carbs: 15g, Protein: 5g, Sugar: 0g

6. WATERMELON CUCUMBER BITES

P.T.: 10 min

C.T.: 0 min

M.C.: Assembly

SERVINGS: 4

INGR.:

1/2 watermelon, cut into 1-inch cubes

1 cucumber, sliced into rounds

1/4 cup feta cheese, crumbled

2 Tblsp balsamic glaze

Fresh mint for garnish

DIRECTIONS:

Assemble by placing a cucumber round on a watermelon cube.

Top with crumbled feta and a drizzle of balsamic glaze.

Garnish with a small mint leaf.

TIPS:

For a party snack, skewer the watermelon, cucumber, and feta onto toothpicks.

Chill the ingredients before assembly for a refreshing snack.

N.V.: Calories: 70, Fat: 2g, Carbs: 11g, Protein: 2g, Sugar: 9g

CHAPTER 8: VEGETARIAN AND VEGAN OPTIONS
PLANT-BASED HIGH-CARB MEALS

1. QUINOA AND BLACK BEAN BURRITO BOWL

P.T.: 15 min
C.T.: 25 min
M.C.: Boiling & Sauteing
SERVINGS: 4
INGR.:
1 cup quinoa
2 cups water
1 can (15 oz) black beans, drained and rinsed
1 cup corn kernels, fresh or frozen
1 avocado, diced
1 cup cherry tomatoes, halved
1/2 red onion, finely chopped
1/4 cup fresh cilantro, chopped
Juice of 1 lime
Salt and pepper to taste
1 tsp cumin
1 tsp paprika
DIRECTIONS:
Rinse quinoa under cold water. In a medium pot, combine quinoa and water. Bring to a boil, then cover and reduce to a simmer for 15 minutes, or until water is absorbed. Remove from heat and let sit, covered, for 5 minutes.

In a large bowl, mix cooked quinoa with black beans, corn, avocado, cherry tomatoes, red onion, cilantro, lime juice, cumin, paprika, salt, and pepper.

Serve chilled or at room temperature, adjusting seasoning as desired.

TIPS:
Drizzle with a tangy yogurt sauce for added flavor.

Top with roasted sweet potatoes for extra heartiness.

N.V.: Calories: 320, Fat: 9g, Carbs: 50g, Protein: 12g, Sugar: 3g

2. VEGAN LENTIL BOLOGNESE

P.T.: 10 min
C.T.: 45 min
M.C.: Sauteing & Simmering
SERVINGS: 4
INGR.:
1 cup green lentils, rinsed
1 Tblsp olive oil
1 onion, diced
2 cloves garlic, minced
1 carrot, diced
1 stalk celery, diced
1 can (28 oz) crushed tomatoes
2 Tblsp tomato paste
1 tsp oregano
1 tsp basil
Salt and pepper to taste
1/4 tsp red pepper flakes (optional)
Whole wheat or gluten-free pasta, cooked
DIRECTIONS:
In a large pan, heat olive oil over medium

heat. Add onion, garlic, carrot, and celery. Saute until softened, about 5 minutes.

Add lentils, crushed tomatoes, tomato paste, oregano, basil, salt, pepper, and red pepper flakes. Stir to combine.

Bring to a boil, then reduce heat and simmer for 30-35 minutes, or until lentils are tender and sauce has thickened.

Serve over cooked pasta of your choice.

TIPS:

Add a splash of red wine for depth of flavor during cooking.

Garnish with nutritional yeast for a cheesy flavor.

N.V.: Calories: 380, Fat: 5g, Carbs: 65g, Protein: 20g, Sugar: 12g

3. SWEET POTATO AND CHICKPEA CURRY

P.T.: 15 min
C.T.: 30 min
M.C.: Simmering
SERVINGS: 4
INGR.:

2 large sweet potatoes, peeled and cubed
1 can (15 oz) chickpeas, drained and rinsed
1 onion, diced
2 cloves garlic, minced
1 Tblsp ginger, grated
1 can (14 oz) coconut milk
1 Tblsp curry powder
1 tsp turmeric
Salt to taste
1 Tblsp olive oil
Fresh cilantro for garnish
Cooked rice, for serving

DIRECTIONS:

Heat olive oil in a large pot over medium heat. Add onion, garlic, and ginger. Saute until onion is translucent.

Add curry powder and turmeric, stirring for about 1 minute until fragrant.

Add sweet potatoes, chickpeas, and coconut milk. Bring to a boil, then cover, reduce heat, and simmer for 20-25 minutes or until sweet potatoes are tender.

Season with salt to taste. Serve over rice and garnish with fresh cilantro.

TIPS:

Squeeze lime juice over the curry before serving for added zing.

Incorporate spinach or kale in the last few minutes of cooking for extra greens.

N.V.: Calories: 420, Fat: 18g, Carbs: 55g, Protein: 10g, Sugar: 9g

4. HIGH-CARB VEGAN PIZZA

P.T.: 20 min
C.T.: 15 min
M.C.: Baking
SERVINGS: 2

INGR.:

1 pre-made pizza crust, whole wheat
1/2 cup tomato sauce
1 cup spinach leaves

1/2 bell pepper, sliced

1/4 red onion, thinly sliced

1/2 cup canned artichoke hearts, drained and chopped

1/4 cup black olives, sliced

1/4 cup vegan cheese shreds (optional)

1 tsp oregano

1 tsp basil

Chili flakes to taste

DIRECTIONS:

Preheat oven according to pizza crust package instructions.

Spread tomato sauce evenly over the crust.

Top with spinach, bell pepper, red onion, artichoke hearts, black olives, and vegan cheese.

Sprinkle with oregano, basil, and chili flakes.

Bake according to crust instructions, or until edges are golden and toppings are heated through.

TIPS:

Add sliced mushrooms or zucchini for extra veggies.

Drizzle with balsamic glaze before serving for a gourmet touch.

N.V.: Calories: 350, Fat: 9g, Carbs: 55g, Protein: 12g, Sugar: 8g

LOW-CARB VEGETARIAN DELIGHTS

1. ZUCCHINI NOODLES WITH AVOCADO PESTO

P.T.: 10 min

C.T.: 0 min

M.C.: No cook

SERVINGS: 2

INGR.:

2 large zucchinis

1 ripe avocado

1/2 cup fresh basil leaves

2 cloves garlic

2 Tblsp lemon juice

1/4 cup pine nuts

Salt and pepper to taste

Cherry tomatoes for garnish

DIRECTIONS:

Use a spiralizer to create noodles from the zucchinis. Place them in a large bowl.

In a food processor, blend the avocado, basil, garlic, lemon juice, pine nuts, salt, and pepper until smooth.

Toss the zucchini noodles with the avocado pesto until well coated. Serve garnished with cherry tomatoes.

TIPS:

For added protein, top with toasted chickpeas.

Chill before serving for a refreshing meal.

N.V.: Calories: 250, Fat: 20g, Carbs: 18g, Protein: 6g, Sugar: 5g

2. CAULIFLOWER RICE STIR-FRY

P.T.: 15 min
C.T.: 10 min
M.C.: Sautéing
SERVINGS: 4
INGR.:
1 head cauliflower, grated into 'rice'
1 Tblsp sesame oil
1 small onion, diced
1 cup mixed vegetables (carrots, peas, bell peppers)
2 cloves garlic, minced
1 Tblsp soy sauce
Salt and pepper to taste
2 green onions, sliced for garnish
Sesame seeds for garnish
DIRECTIONS:
Heat sesame oil in a large skillet over medium heat. Add onion and garlic, sauté until soft.
Increase heat to medium-high, add mixed vegetables, and cook for 2-3 minutes.
Add cauliflower rice, soy sauce, salt, and pepper. Stir-fry for 5-7 minutes or until cauliflower is tender.
Garnish with green onions and sesame seeds before serving.
TIPS:
Add a scrambled egg or tofu for extra protein.
Adjust the seasoning with additional soy sauce or a splash of chili sauce for heat.
N.V.: Calories: 120, Fat: 4g, Carbs: 18g, Protein: 4g, Sugar: 6g

3. MUSHROOM AND SPINACH OMELETTE

P.T.: 5 min
C.T.: 10 min
M.C.: Frying
SERVINGS: 1
INGR.:
2 large eggs
1 cup spinach, washed and chopped
1/2 cup mushrooms, sliced
1 Tblsp olive oil
Salt and pepper to taste
1/4 cup shredded cheese (optional for vegan, can use dairy-free cheese)
DIRECTIONS:
Heat olive oil in a skillet over medium heat.
Add mushrooms, cooking until they are soft.
Add spinach and cook until wilted.
Beat eggs with salt and pepper, then pour over the spinach and mushrooms. Cook until the eggs are set, fold the omelette in half.
If using cheese, sprinkle it over the omelette before folding. Serve immediately.
TIPS:
Enhance the flavor with fresh herbs like chives or parsley.
Serve with a side of avocado for healthy fats.
N.V.: Calories: 220, Fat: 18g, Carbs: 3g, Protein: 13g, Sugar: 1g

VEGAN SNACKS AND DESSERTS

1. VEGAN CHOCOLATE AVOCADO TRUFFLES

P.T.: 15 min
C.T.: 0 min (Requires 1 hr chilling)
M.C.: No cook
SERVINGS: 12 truffles
INGR.:
2 ripe avocados
1/2 cup cocoa powder, plus extra for coating
1/4 cup maple syrup
1 tsp vanilla extract
Pinch of salt

DIRECTIONS:
Mash the avocados in a bowl until smooth. Mix in cocoa powder, maple syrup, vanilla extract, and a pinch of salt until well combined.
Refrigerate the mixture for 1 hour to firm up. Scoop out and roll into balls, then coat with additional cocoa powder.

TIPS:
Keep truffles refrigerated until serving.
Experiment with coatings, such as crushed nuts or coconut flakes, for variety.

N.V.: Calories: 80, Fat: 5g, Carbs: 10g, Protein: 2g, Sugar: 5g

2. VEGAN BANANA NUT MUFFINS

P.T.: 10 min
C.T.: 20 min
M.C.: Baking
SERVINGS: 12 muffins
INGR.:
3 ripe bananas, mashed
1/4 cup vegetable oil
1/4 cup almond milk
1/2 cup maple syrup
1 tsp vanilla extract
2 cups whole wheat flour
1 tsp baking soda
1/2 tsp salt
1/2 cup walnuts, chopped

DIRECTIONS:
Preheat oven to 350°F (175°C) and line a muffin tin with paper liners.
Mix bananas, oil, almond milk, maple syrup, and vanilla in a bowl.
Combine flour, baking soda, and salt in another bowl. Gradually add to the wet ingredients, stirring until just combined. Fold in walnuts.
Divide batter among muffin cups and bake for 20 minutes or until a toothpick comes out clean.

TIPS:
Add a sprinkle of cinnamon or nutmeg to the batter for extra flavor.
Substitute walnuts with pecans or chocolate chips if desired.

N.V.: Calories: 200, Fat: 8g, Carbs: 30g, Protein: 4g, Sugar: 12g

3. CRISPY KALE CHIPS

P.T.: 5 min

C.T.: 15 min

M.C.: Baking

SERVINGS: 4

INGR.:

1 bunch kale, stems removed and leaves torn

1 Tblsp olive oil

Salt to taste

DIRECTIONS:

Preheat oven to 350°F (175°C). Line a baking sheet with parchment paper.

Toss kale leaves with olive oil and salt. Spread on the baking sheet in a single layer.

Bake for 15 minutes, or until crisp.

TIPS:

Ensure kale is dry before adding oil for the crispiest result.

Experiment with seasonings like nutritional yeast, garlic powder, or smoked paprika.

N.V.: Calories: 58, Fat: 3.5g, Carbs: 6g, Protein: 2g, Sugar: 0g

CHAPTER 9: QUICK AND EASY RECIPES
15-MINUTE BREAKFASTS

1. AVOCADO TOAST WITH POACHED EGG

P.T.: 5 min
C.T.: 10 min
M.C.: Toasting & Poaching
SERVINGS: 2
INGR.:
2 slices whole grain bread
1 ripe avocado
2 eggs
Salt and pepper to taste
Red pepper flakes, optional
1 Tblsp white vinegar (for poaching eggs)

DIRECTIONS:
Toast the bread slices to your preference. Mash the avocado in a bowl, season with salt and pepper. Spread the mashed avocado evenly on the toasted bread slices.

To poach the eggs, bring a pot of water to a simmer and add the vinegar. Crack each egg into a small bowl and gently slide them into the simmering water. Poach for 3-4 minutes for soft yolks. Remove with a slotted spoon and drain on paper towels.

Place a poached egg on each avocado toast. Season with salt, pepper, and red pepper flakes if desired.

TIPS:
For added flavor, top with chopped fresh herbs like cilantro or parsley.

Serve with a side of mixed greens for a complete breakfast.

N.V.: Calories: 300, Fat: 20g, Carbs: 23g, Protein: 13g, Sugar: 3g

2. BERRY AND YOGURT SMOOTHIE

P.T.: 5 min
C.T.: 0 min
M.C.: Blending
SERVINGS: 2
INGR.:
1 cup frozen mixed berries (strawberries, blueberries, raspberries)
1 banana
1 cup low-fat Greek yogurt
1/2 cup almond milk
1 Tblsp honey, optional
1/2 tsp vanilla extract

DIRECTIONS:
In a blender, combine the frozen berries, banana, Greek yogurt, almond milk, honey (if using), and vanilla extract.

Blend until smooth. If the smoothie is too thick, add more almond milk until you reach your desired consistency.

Serve immediately, garnished with a few whole berries on top.

TIPS:
Freeze the banana ahead of time for an extra cold and creamy texture.

Add a scoop of protein powder for an extra protein boost.

N.V.: Calories: 180, Fat: 2g, Carbs: 30g, Protein: 10g, Sugar: 18g

3. SPINACH AND FETA MICROWAVE MUG OMELETTE

P.T.: 2 min
C.T.: 3 min
M.C.: Microwaving
SERVINGS: 1
INGR.:
2 eggs
1/4 cup fresh spinach, chopped
2 Tblsp feta cheese, crumbled
Salt and pepper to taste
1 Tblsp milk (any kind)
Butter or oil (for greasing the mug)

DIRECTIONS:
Grease the inside of a microwave-safe mug with butter or oil.

In the mug, beat the eggs with milk, salt, and pepper. Stir in the chopped spinach and crumbled feta cheese.

Microwave on high for 1 minute. Stir, then microwave for another 1-2 minutes, or until the eggs are set.

Let the mug omelette stand for a minute before eating. Serve straight from the mug or slide it onto a plate.

TIPS:
Customize your mug omelette with additional ingredients like diced tomatoes, onions, or cooked bacon bits.

Watch the omelette closely as it cooks, as microwave powers can vary. Adjust cooking time accordingly to avoid overcooking.

N.V.: Calories: 200, Fat: 14g, Carbs: 2g, Protein: 16g, Sugar: 1g

QUICK LUNCHES FOR BUSY DAYS

1. CHICKPEA SALAD SANDWICH

P.T.: 10 min
C.T.: 0 min
M.C.: No cook
SERVINGS: 2
INGR.:
1 can (15 oz) chickpeas, drained and rinsed
2 Tblsp vegan mayonnaise
1 Tblsp mustard
1/4 cup celery, finely chopped
1/4 cup red onion, finely chopped
Salt and pepper to taste
4 slices whole grain bread
Lettuce leaves

DIRECTIONS:
In a bowl, mash the chickpeas with a fork. Mix in vegan mayonnaise, mustard, celery, red onion, salt, and pepper until well combined.

Spread the chickpea mixture on two slices of bread. Add lettuce leaves, then top with the remaining slices of bread to make sandwiches.

TIPS:

Add a dash of paprika or curry powder to the chickpea mixture for extra flavor.

For a gluten-free option, serve the chickpea salad over a bed of greens instead of bread.

N.V.: Calories: 350, Fat: 9g, Carbs: 52g, Protein: 15g, Sugar: 7g

2. AVOCADO & QUINOA SALAD

P.T.: 5 min
C.T.: 15 min
M.C.: Boiling
SERVINGS: 2
INGR.:
1 cup quinoa, rinsed
2 cups water
1 ripe avocado, diced
1/2 cup cherry tomatoes, halved
1/4 cup cucumber, diced
2 Tblsp lemon juice
Salt and pepper to taste
2 Tblsp olive oil
Fresh cilantro, for garnish
DIRECTIONS:

In a medium saucepan, bring quinoa and water to a boil. Reduce heat to low, cover, and simmer for 15 minutes, or until quinoa is fluffy and water is absorbed. Let it cool.

In a large bowl, combine cooled quinoa, diced avocado, cherry tomatoes, cucumber, lemon juice, salt, pepper, and olive oil. Toss gently.

Serve garnished with fresh cilantro.

TIPS:

Chill the salad for 30 minutes before serving for a refreshing touch.

Add a sprinkle of feta cheese or olives for extra flavor.

N.V.: Calories: 480, Fat: 22g, Carbs: 62g, Protein: 12g, Sugar: 3g

3. TURKEY & SPINACH WRAP

P.T.: 5 min
C.T.: 0 min
M.C.: Wrapping
SERVINGS: 2
INGR.:
2 whole wheat tortillas
4 slices turkey breast
1 cup spinach leaves
1/4 cup shredded carrots
2 Tblsp hummus

Salt and pepper to taste

DIRECTIONS:

Lay out the tortillas on a flat surface. Spread 1 Tblsp of hummus on each tortilla.

Place two slices of turkey breast on each tortilla, followed by a layer of spinach leaves and shredded carrots. Season with salt and pepper.

Roll up the tortillas tightly, cut in half, and serve.

TIPS:

For a vegetarian version, substitute turkey with sliced avocado or additional veggies.

Serve with a side of yogurt or fresh fruit for a complete meal.

N.V.: Calories: 320, Fat: 9g, Carbs: 35g, Protein: 25g, Sugar: 5g

SPEEDY DINNERS

1. PAN-SEARED SALMON WITH AVOCADO SALSA

P.T.: 5 min
C.T.: 10 min
M.C.: Pan-searing
SERVINGS: 2
INGR.:

2 salmon fillets (6 oz each)
1 Tblsp olive oil
Salt and pepper to taste

For the Avocado Salsa:

1 ripe avocado, diced
1/2 red onion, finely chopped
Juice of 1 lime
1 Tblsp cilantro, chopped
Salt to taste

DIRECTIONS:

Season the salmon fillets with salt and pepper. Heat olive oil in a skillet over medium-high heat. Place salmon skin-side up and cook for 5 minutes, then flip and cook for another 4-5 minutes until desired doneness.

For the salsa, combine avocado, red onion, lime juice, cilantro, and salt in a bowl.

Serve the salmon with avocado salsa on top.

TIPS:

Ensure the skillet is hot before adding the salmon for a crispy skin.

Add diced tomatoes to the salsa for extra freshness.

N.V.: Calories: 400, Fat: 28g, Carbs: 8g, Protein: 34g, Sugar: 2g

2. CHICKPEA AND SPINACH STIR-FRY

P.T.: 5 min
C.T.: 10 min
M.C.: Stir-frying
SERVINGS: 2
INGR.:

1 can (15 oz) chickpeas, drained and rinsed
2 cups spinach leaves
1 garlic clove, minced
2 Tblsp olive oil
1 tsp cumin
Salt and pepper to taste
Lemon wedges for serving

DIRECTIONS:

Heat olive oil in a pan over medium heat. Add garlic and sauté for 1 minute.

Add chickpeas and cumin, cook for 5 minutes until chickpeas are golden.

Add spinach and cook until wilted. Season with salt and pepper.

Serve with lemon wedges on the side.

TIPS:

For a complete meal, serve over quinoa or brown rice.

Add a pinch of chili flakes for a spicy kick.

N.V.: Calories: 295, Fat: 14g, Carbs: 34g, Protein: 10g, Sugar: 6g

3. QUICK VEGGIE PASTA

P.T.: 5 min
C.T.: 10 min
M.C.: Boiling
SERVINGS: 2
INGR.:

8 oz whole wheat pasta

2 cups mixed vegetables (broccoli, bell peppers, peas)

2 garlic cloves, minced

2 Tblsp olive oil

Salt and pepper to taste

Grated Parmesan cheese (optional)

DIRECTIONS:

Cook pasta according to package instructions, adding mixed vegetables to the boiling water during the last 3 minutes of cooking. Drain.

In the same pot, heat olive oil over medium heat. Add garlic and sauté until fragrant.

Add the cooked pasta and vegetables back into the pot. Toss to combine. Season with salt and pepper.

Serve with grated Parmesan cheese if desired.

TIPS:

Customize with your favorite vegetables or whatever you have on hand.

Add red pepper flakes for extra heat.

N.V.: Calories: 350, Fat: 14g, Carbs: 48g, Protein: 12g, Sugar: 4g

SIMPLE SNACKS

1. APPLE SLICES WITH PEANUT BUTTER

P.T.: 5 min
C.T.: 0 min
M.C.: No cook
SERVINGS: 2
INGR.:

2 large apples

4 Tblsp natural peanut butter

A pinch of cinnamon (optional)

DIRECTIONS:

Core and slice the apples into thin pieces.

Spread each apple slice with peanut butter.

Sprinkle a pinch of cinnamon over the slices for added flavor.

TIPS:

For a crunchy twist, add granola on top of the peanut butter before serving.

Swap peanut butter with almond butter for variety.

N.V.: Calories: 210, Fat: 12g, Carbs: 24g, Protein: 5g, Sugar: 16g

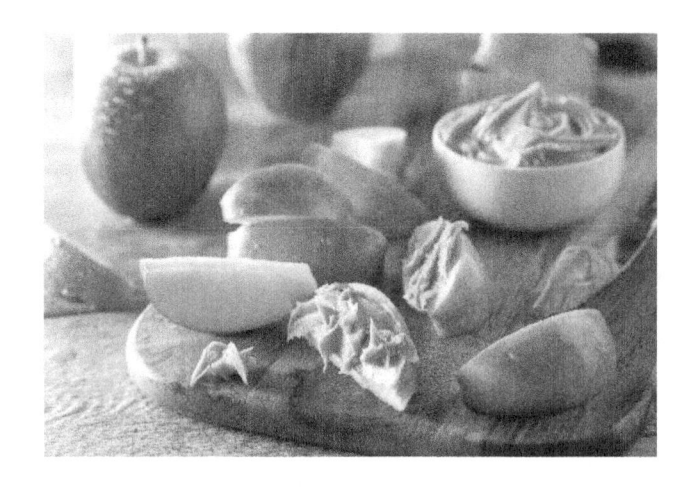

2. GREEK YOGURT AND HONEY PARFAIT

P.T.: 5 min

C.T.: 0 min

M.C.: Layering

SERVINGS: 2

INGR.:

2 cups Greek yogurt, low-fat

4 Tblsp honey

1/2 cup granola

1/2 cup mixed berries

DIRECTIONS:

In two serving glasses, layer Greek yogurt, honey, granola, and mixed berries.

Repeat the layers until the glasses are filled. Serve immediately.

TIPS:

For added texture, include nuts or seeds with the granola layer.

Layer with seasonal fruits for variety throughout the year.

N.V.: Calories: 320, Fat: 4g, Carbs: 55g, Protein: 20g, Sugar: 35g

3. HUMMUS AND VEGGIE STICKS

P.T.: 5 min

C.T.: 0 min

M.C.: No cook

SERVINGS: 2

INGR.:

1 cup hummus

1 carrot, peeled and cut into sticks

1 cucumber, cut into sticks

1 bell pepper, cut into sticks

DIRECTIONS:

Arrange the hummus in a small bowl for dipping.

Surround the bowl with an assortment of carrot, cucumber, and bell pepper sticks.

TIPS:

For a spicy twist, sprinkle paprika over the hummus.

Serve with whole grain pita bread for an extra filling snack.

N.V.: Calories: 180, Fat: 9g, Carbs: 20g, Protein: 8g, Sugar: 5g

CHAPTER 10: THE 45-DAY CARB CYCLING MEAL PLAN

WEEK 1-6: DAILY MEAL PLANS

Week 1-2

Day	Breakfast	Lunch	Dinner
Monday	Oatmeal banana berry bake	Quinoa power salad	Roasted vegetable and farro bowl
Tuesday	Sweet potato and black bean breakfast burritos	Sweet potato lentil bowl	Lemon herb chicken pasta
Wednesday	Mango chia pudding parfait	Chickpea avocado wrap	Balsamic glazed salmon with quinoa and spinach
Thursday	Peanut butter and jelly oatmeal	Turkey and quinoa stuffed peppers	Thai peanut sweet potato buddha bowl
Friday	Spinach and feta breakfast quiche	Asian chicken salad	Mushroom risotto with peas
Saturday	Blueberry almond pancakes	Mediterranean lentil pasta salad	Creamy coconut lentil curry
Sunday	Spinach and feta omelette	Avocado and egg breakfast bowl	Smoked salmon and cream cheese roll-ups

Week 3-4

Day	Breakfast	Lunch	Dinner
Monday	High protein hemp oatmeal	Vegetarian chili with quinoa	Pumpkin and sweet potato soup
Tuesday	Mixed berry smoothie bowl	Sweet corn and black bean salad	Lentil and mushroom stew
Wednesday	Chia seed and berry parfait	Zucchini and carrot noodles with pesto	Veggie pasta with tomato sauce
Thursday	Avocado and poached egg toast	Cauliflower rice stir fry	Grilled chicken with asparagus
Friday	Coconut yogurt with nuts and seeds	Spinach and goat cheese salad	Shrimp and avocado salad
Saturday	Scrambled tofu with spinach	Broccoli and cheddar stuffed peppers	Eggplant lasagna with spinach
Sunday	Keto avocado smoothie	Avocado chicken salad	Salmon and roasted vegetables

Week 5-6

Day	Breakfast	Lunch	Dinner
Monday	Vegan blueberry muffins	Black bean soup	Quinoa stuffed bell peppers
Tuesday	Tofu scramble with veggies	Vegetable stir-fry with brown rice	Mediterranean vegetable pasta
Wednesday	Berry quinoa breakfast bowl	Curried lentil soup	Chickpea and spinach curry
Thursday	Almond butter smoothie	Greek salad with tofu	Zucchini noodles with avocado pesto
Friday	Keto berry parfait	Chicken caesar salad	Baked salmon with steamed broccoli
Saturday	Spinach and mushroom egg muffins	Tuna salad lettuce wraps	Stuffed avocados with chicken and walnuts
Sunday	Low carb coconut pancakes	Grilled vegetable platter	Eggplant pizza

ADJUSTING THE PLAN TO YOUR NEEDS

Understanding Your Body's Signals

The first step in customizing this plan is to listen—really listen—to your body. Your body communicates in subtle ways, hinting when it needs more energy, signaling when it's satisfied, and showing signs of progress or stagnation. If you find yourself feeling sluggish on low-carb days, it might be a cue to slightly increase your carb intake, especially if you're engaging in heavy workouts. Conversely, if high-carb days make you feel bloated or slow, consider reducing the carbs a bit and observe how you feel.

Adapting to Physical Activity

Physical activity significantly influences how your body utilizes carbs. On days filled with intense workouts, your body can benefit from higher carb intake to replenish glycogen stores and aid recovery. These are the days when adding a serving of quinoa or sweet potato to your meals can be particularly beneficial. On the flip side, sedentary days require less energy, making low-carb meals more appropriate. The key is to align your carb intake with your activity level, ensuring your body gets what it needs, when it needs it.

Balancing Meals with Real Life

Life's unpredictability calls for flexibility in your meal plan. Social events, family gatherings, and work commitments often come unannounced. When these situations arise, give yourself grace. If you find yourself at a birthday party on a low-carb day, it's okay to partake in a slice of cake. What's important is getting back on track with the next meal, not letting a single deviation derail your entire plan.

Incorporating Variety

Variety isn't just the spice of life; it's a crucial component of a sustainable meal plan. Eating the same meals repeatedly can lead to boredom and nutritional gaps. To keep things interesting and balanced, regularly introduce new recipes and swap out ingredients in existing ones. Experiment with different vegetables, proteins, and healthy fats to discover new flavors and textures. This not only makes your meals more enjoyable but also ensures a wider range of nutrients.

Listening to Hunger and Fullness Cues

One of the most empowering aspects of carb cycling is learning to tune into your body's hunger and fullness signals. Carb cycling isn't about strict calorie counting or rigid meal schedules. It's about eating when you're hungry and stopping when you're satisfied. Some days you might find yourself hungrier than usual, and that's okay. Allow yourself to eat a little more, focusing on nutrient-dense foods that satisfy and nourish. Other days, you might not feel as hungry, and that's also fine. Learning to trust your body's cues is a powerful step toward a healthier relationship with food.

Adjusting for Weight Loss or Gain

Your carb cycling plan can be adjusted to support weight loss, maintenance, or gain, depending on your goals. If you're looking to lose weight, you might incorporate an additional low-carb day or reduce the portion sizes on high-carb days. For weight gain, particularly muscle mass, increasing the portion sizes on high-carb days and ensuring adequate protein intake can be effective. Remember, changes should be gradual and always in tune with how your body responds.

Mindful Eating Practices

How you eat is just as important as what you eat. Adopting mindful eating practices—such as eating without distractions, chewing thoroughly, and savoring each bite—can enhance your meal plan's effectiveness. Mindful eating helps in recognizing satiety cues, enjoying your meals more fully, and digesting your food better. It turns each meal into an opportunity for mindfulness and gratitude, enriching your carb cycling journey beyond mere nutrition.

Hydration and Sleep

Never underestimate the power of hydration and sleep in supporting your carb cycling plan. Drinking adequate water aids digestion, nutrient absorption, and appetite regulation. Meanwhile, quality sleep supports hormonal balance, recovery, and overall well-being. Both are foundational elements that amplify the benefits of your meal plan.

Community and Support

Embarking on a nutritional plan can be challenging, but you don't have to do it alone. Sharing your journey with friends, family, or online communities can provide support, accountability, and motivation. Whether it's swapping recipes, sharing successes, or navigating challenges together, a supportive community can make all the difference.

Flexibility is Key

Finally, remember that flexibility is key. Life is dynamic, and so are your body's needs. Be willing to adjust your meal plan as you go, based on how you feel, your activity levels, and life's inevitable ebbs and flows. The goal of the 45-day carb cycling plan is not to follow a rigid set of rules but to learn, adapt, and ultimately find a balanced way of eating that supports your health, happiness, and well-being.

Tracking Your Progress

Journaling is more than just a record-keeping exercise; it's a dialogue with oneself. Begin each day by jotting down your starting point your weight, how you feel, and perhaps a quick note on your sleep quality from the night before. As your day unfolds, keep a log of your meals, noting not just what you eat but how those foods make you feel. Do certain meals leave you energized and satisfied, or sluggish and craving more? This insight is golden, as it helps tailor the meal plan to your body's unique needs.

While metrics such as weight and body measurements offer tangible markers of progress, they don't tell the whole story. Your energy levels, strength, mood, and how your clothes fit are equally, if not more, important indicators of your journey's success. Celebrate these non-scale victories as they come, for they are true reflections of your body's positive response to the carb cycling plan.

Sometimes, the mirror reflects what our minds want to see, and the scale can be an unreliable narrator of our progress. This is where photos can be incredibly telling. Taking weekly photos from multiple angles can provide an objective view of the physical changes happening in your body. These snapshots serve as a powerful motivational tool, clearly showing where you've come from and where you're heading.

As you progress through the 45-day plan, your body will start to communicate with you in new ways. Perhaps you'll notice certain carbs make you feel more energized than others, or that your body responds particularly well to certain types of exercise on high-carb days. This feedback is precious, guiding you to fine-tune your meal plan and workout regimen to harness the most benefit.

Setting goals at the outset is crucial, but so is the willingness to revise them. As you progress, you might find some goals were too ambitious, while others were too modest. Adjusting your goals doesn't mean you're off track; it means you're becoming more attuned to your body and what's achievable. It's a sign of growth.

Sharing your goals and progress with someone you trust can significantly enhance your journey. Whether it's a friend, family member, or an online community, having someone to celebrate your victories with, and who can offer encouragement during challenging times, can make all the difference. Accountability doesn't mean handing over your autonomy; it means expanding your support network.

Every step forward deserves recognition. Completed your first week? Celebrate it. Noticed improvements in your stamina or strength? Give yourself a pat on the back. These milestones, no matter how small they may seem, are stepping stones towards your larger goal. Celebrating them keeps the journey joyful and rewarding.

At the journey's end, take time to reflect on the path you've traversed. What worked for you? What challenges did you face, and how did you overcome them? This reflection isn't just about acknowledging your hard work and achievements; it's about gleaning lessons that you can carry forward, beyond the 45 days.

MEASUREMENT CONVERSION TABLE

Volume Conversions

Measurement	US Standard	Metric
1 teaspoon (tsp)	1 tsp	5 milliliters (mL)
1 tablespoon (Tblsp)	1 Tblsp	15 mL
1 fluid ounce (fl oz)	1 fl oz	30 mL
1 cup	1 cup	240 mL
1 pint (pt)	1 pt	473 mL
1 quart (qt)	1 qt	946 mL
1 gallon (gal)	1 gal	3.785 liters (L)

Weight Conversions

Measurement	US Standard	Metric
1 ounce (oz)	1 oz	28 grams (g)
1 pound (lb)	1 lb	454 g

Length Conversions

Measurement	US Standard	Metric
1 inch (in)	1 in	2.54 centimeters (cm)

CHAPTER 11: BEYOND THE PLATE
COMPLEMENTING CARB CYCLING WITH EXERCISE

Imagine your body as an instrument. Nutrition tunes this instrument, while exercise plays the melody. Together, they create harmony. Carb cycling, with its rhythm of high and low carb days, acts as the sheet music for this melody, guiding your body's energy use and replenishment. Exercise, then, varies the tempo and intensity, from the gentle adagio of yoga to the vivacious allegro of high-intensity interval training (HIIT). The beauty of combining carb cycling and exercise lies in their mutual support. On high-carb days, when your body is flush with energy, it's the perfect time to engage in high-intensity activities that demand more glycogen, such as weight lifting, sprinting, or intense aerobic classes. These exercises capitalize on the available energy, fueling powerful workouts that stimulate muscle growth and fat loss. Conversely, low-carb days invite a gentler approach. Think of these days as your body's adagio movement, where the pace slows but the depth of the music deepens. Gentle yoga, leisurely walks, or light cycling allow your body to burn fat without depleting it, harmonizing with the lower energy intake. Muscle is the maestro of metabolism, conducting the rate at which your body burns energy. Incorporating resistance training into your routine not only builds muscle mass but also enhances your metabolic tempo, allowing your body to burn more calories, even in repose. On your high-carb days, engage in strength training to feed your muscles the energy they crave for growth and repair. Cardiovascular exercise, with its myriad forms, adds versatility to your melody. High-intensity cardio sessions are splendidly suited to high-carb days, turning the body's fuel into fiery workouts that improve heart health and endurance. On low-carb days, low-intensity steady-state (LISS) cardio complements the body's fuel strategy, efficiently burning fat in a flame fueled by oxygen and patience. Rest and recovery are the silences between the notes that make the music of your movement meaningful. Incorporating flexibility and recovery practices, such as stretching, foam rolling, or meditation, especially on low-carb days, supports muscle repair, reduces the risk of injury, and prepares your body to return to the allegro of high-carb days with vigor. The most profound music is not found in the notes themselves but in how they resonate with the listener. Similarly, the most effective exercise regimen is not prescriptive but adaptive, listening to the body's responses, adjusting the intensity, and embracing rest as readily as activity. Pay attention to how your body feels during workouts on different days and adjust accordingly. Some days, it may sing with strength, while on others, it may whisper for rest. Exercise and carb cycling play a duet that also uplifts the mind and spirit. The variety in workout intensity and dietary intake keeps both the body and mind engaged, warding off the monotony that can dampen motivation. The achievement of pushing through a tough workout or the calm of a restorative yoga session adds layers of satisfaction and accomplishment to the carb cycling journey. Just as music is meant to be shared, so too is the journey of health and wellness. Engage with a community of like-minded individuals who are also navigating the harmonies of carb cycling and exercise. Share successes, challenges, and tips. The support and inspiration found in a community can be the chorus that uplifts you through the challenging movements of your health symphony. Complementing carb cycling with exercise is about more than just physical health; it's a holistic approach to living fully. It's about finding joy in the foods you eat and the movement you choose. It's about tuning into your body's needs and responding with care. This journey is personal, dynamic, and ever-evolving, much like a life-long love affair with a melody that grows with you, note by note, step by step.

MINDFULNESS AND MENTAL HEALTH

In the landscape of wellness, where the terrain is as much mental as it is physical, mindfulness stands as a beacon, illuminating the path to mental health. Beyond the plate, beyond the gym, lies the vast expanse of our inner selves—a domain where thoughts swirl like leaves in an autumn wind, where emotions ebb and flow like the tides. It's here, in the quietude of our minds, that the essence of health is nurtured, where the seeds of mindfulness can bloom into a garden of tranquility. Mindfulness, in its essence, is the art of being present. It's the practice of anchoring ourselves in the now, embracing each moment with acceptance and without judgment. In the context of carb cycling and overall wellness, mindfulness transforms the journey from a mere series of dietary choices and exercises into a holistic voyage of self-discovery and growth. Mindfulness begins where most things in nutrition do—at the plate. Eating mindfully is not just about what we eat, but how we eat. It's about savoring each bite, recognizing the flavors, textures, and aromas of our food, and acknowledging the nourishment it provides. This practice turns each meal into a meditation, a moment of gratitude for the earth's bounty and the effort that brought it to our table. Mindful eating slows us down, allowing our bodies to recognize satiety cues, reducing the likelihood of overeating, and enhancing our relationship with food. Breath, the most fundamental rhythm of life, is also a bridge to mindfulness. In moments of stress, anxiety, or disconnection, focusing on the breath can be a powerful tool to anchor ourselves in the present. Simple breathing techniques, such as deep diaphragmatic breathing, can calm the mind, reduce stress, and improve cognitive function, making us more attuned to our bodies' needs and better equipped to make healthful choices. Our bodies speak, but too often, we don't listen. Mindfulness strengthens the mind-body connection, enabling us to hear what our bodies are telling us. Whether it's hunger, fullness, fatigue, or the need for movement, mindfulness encourages a dialogue with our bodies. By listening, we learn to respond with kindness, giving our bodies what they need—be it nourishment, rest, or activity—thereby supporting our physical health and emotional well-being. Mindfulness fosters compassion—towards ourselves and others. Embarking on a journey of health and wellness is a courageous act, one that is inevitably met with challenges and setbacks. Mindfulness teaches us to meet these moments with compassion, to greet our perceived failures not with judgment or self-criticism, but with kindness and understanding. This self-compassion is the foundation upon which resilience is built, enabling us to persevere, to learn from our experiences, and to continue on our path with renewed vigor. In a world that prizes constant motion, stillness is often overlooked. Yet, it's in stillness that we find clarity. Mindfulness encourages us to find moments of stillness in our day, be it through meditation, quiet contemplation, or simply being in nature. These moments of stillness are oases of calm in the desert of our daily lives, providing space for reflection, introspection, and the cultivation of inner peace. Gratitude is the heart of mindfulness, a practice that transforms our perspective, enabling us to see the beauty and bounty in our lives. By cultivating gratitude—for the food on our plate, the ability to move our bodies, the support of our community, and the simple fact of being alive—we enrich our journey, turning each step into an expression of joy and appreciation.

BUILDING A SUPPORTIVE COMMUNITY

A supportive community is a symphony of voices, each unique yet harmoniously intertwined, offering encouragement, empathy, and understanding. It's where triumphs are celebrated with joyous applause and setbacks are met with compassionate hands, lifting you back onto your path. This community becomes your wellness sanctuary—a space where vulnerabilities can be shared without fear of judgment, where questions can be asked and wisdom shared, and where the journey of one becomes the journey of many. In the digital age, the concept of community has transcended geographical boundaries. Online forums, social media platforms, and virtual support groups offer endless possibilities to connect with like-minded individuals embarking on similar health and wellness journeys. Whether it's a carb cycling Facebook group, an Instagram hashtag community, or a forum dedicated to healthy living, these digital spaces allow for the sharing of meal ideas, workout tips, motivational stories, and much more. Yet, the power of local, in-person support groups or fitness classes cannot be understated. The tangible presence of others, the shared sweat and laughter, and the collective energy of in-person gatherings create an indelible bond that digital spaces can complement but not replace. Building a supportive community requires both seeking and cultivating. It involves reaching out, sharing your journey, and in turn, listening and contributing to the journeys of others. It's about celebrating the successes of fellow community members as if they were your own and offering a listening ear or a shoulder to lean on during times of struggle. In this garden of growth, each member is both a gardener and a blossom, nurturing and being nurtured. A community thrives on diversity—the myriad perspectives, experiences, and insights that each member brings to the table enrich the collective wisdom of the group. From the seasoned fitness enthusiast to the novice cook embarking on a health journey, each voice adds depth and dimension to the conversation. This diversity ensures that no matter where you are on your journey, there will always be someone a few steps ahead to guide you and someone a few steps behind whom you can guide. The foundation of a supportive community is a culture of positivity—a shared commitment to uplifting one another and fostering an environment where growth is celebrated, and challenges are met with encouragement. It's about shifting the focus from competition to collaboration, recognizing that the success of one does not diminish the success of another. In this space, each individual's journey is acknowledged as both personal and part of the larger tapestry of the community's collective journey towards wellness. The beauty of a supportive community lies in its ripple effect—the way in which the support, motivation, and inspiration shared within the community extend outward, touching the lives of family members, friends, and even strangers. As you share your journey and the positive impact of the community on your life, you become a beacon of inspiration for others, potentially guiding them towards their own path of health and wellness. At the heart of a supportive community lies empathy and understanding—the ability to put oneself in another's shoes and offer support from a place of genuine understanding and compassion. It's this empathetic connection that creates a safe space for sharing struggles and vulnerabilities, knowing that they will be met with kindness and understanding.

Made in the USA
Las Vegas, NV
10 July 2024